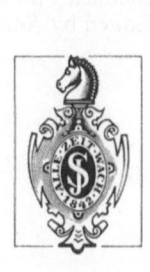

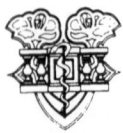 The Bloomsbury Series in Clinical Science

LASERS IN UROLOGY
PRINCIPLES AND PRACTICE

T. A. McNicholas (ed.)

With 63 Figures

Springer-Verlag
London Berlin Heidelberg New York
Paris Tokyo Hong Kong

T. A. McNicholas, MB BS, FRCS
Hunterian Professor, Royal College of Surgeons of England
Senior Registrar, Institute of Urology, St Peter's Group of
Hospitals and The Middlesex Hospital, London WC2, UK

Series Editor
Jack Tinker, BSc, FRCS, FRCP, DIC
Director, Intensive Therapy Unit, The Middlesex Hospital,
London W1N 8AA, UK

Cover illustration: Top: Fig. 2.2 A fibre delivery system (urological system: bare fibre with PTFE cladding); *Inset:* Fig. 3.5. YAG laser fibre coagulating tumours in urethra; *Bottom:* Fig. 1.3. Energy levels in ruby

ISBN-13:978-1-4471-1785-8   e-ISBN-13:978-1-4471-1783-4
DOI:10.1007/978-1-4471-1783-4

British Library Cataloguing in Publication Data
Lasers in urology
1. Medicine. Urology
I. McNicholas, T. A. *1952–* II. Series 616.6

Library of Congress Cataloging-in-Publication Data
Lasers in urology: principles and practice/T. A. McNicholas (ed.). p. cm. —
(The Bloomsbury series in clinical science)

1. Urinary organs—Laser surgery.
I. McNicholas, T. A., 1952– II. Series
[DNLM: 1. Lasers—therapeutic use. 2. Urological Diseases—radiotherapy.
WJ 166 L343] RD571.L38 1990 617.4'61059—dc20
DNLM/DLC   90-9642
for Library of Congress   CIP

Typeset by MJS Publications, Buntingford, Hertfordshire
Printed by Henry Ling, The Dorset Press, Dorchester
2128/3916-543210 Printed on acid-free paper

Series Editor's Foreword

The use of lasers in clinical practice is increasing rapidly, both in the definitive treatment of disease and in the palliation of symptoms. Consequently, this sixth contribution to the Bloomsbury Series in Clinical Science is particularly timely. It opens with an introduction to the basic physics of lasers and then focuses on the current use of lasers in urological practice, and concludes by reflecting on their potential for the future.

Edited, and with several contributions by Tom McNicholas, the book also contains contributions from a number of workers at the National Medical Laser Centre in University College Hospital, London. Given their ever widening application, there can be little doubt that lasers will be a subject the series will return to again.

To date, the series has been concerned with a wide range of topics of fundamental importance in clinical science. It has now gained momentum and future titles continue to reflect its wide sphere of interest. As Series Editor, I would welcome suggestions from readers of topics and issues that could usefully be addressed in the series.

London, May 1990   Jack Tinker

Preface

This monograph reviews urological laser theory and practice. I have been able to call on the assistance of many of my fellow collaborators from the National Medical Laser Centre in Bloomsbury. The members of this multi-specialty group of physicians and surgeons are all engaged in regular clinical laser treatment as well as the fundamental laboratory-based research into the application of laser therapy which is essential for progress and for the more appropriate use of this technology. I am fortunate to be able to draw on the expertise of this, the largest coordinated group of laser workers in Great Britain and probably in Europe, covering all specialties and with a strong bias towards urology. In particular I have taken the opportunity to invite contributions from several authors with practical experience of laser and particularly photodynamic therapy who have now joined the ranks of the National Medical Laser Centre determined to explore in more depth the processes involved before any further clinical application of the techniques, in an effort to improve the quality, reliability and safety of laser therapy in its multiple forms.

Each chapter includes a historical review and a critical review of seminal, crucial or very recent laboratory and clinical work. Chapter 2 gives an overview of "practical lasering", concentrating on the YAG laser as this is the most accessible and immediately useful laser to the urologist. Clinical experience is described in some detail in each chapter, incorporating the practical points we learnt the hard way ourselves. Finally an overall assessment is made of the place of laser treatments in urology and further developments in both the near and far future.

Acknowledgement

The authors would like to thank the Institute of Urology, London, for permission to reproduce the following illustrations: Figs. 3.4, 3.5, 3.6, 4.1, 4.2, 4,3, 4.6, 4.7, 5.4, 5.6, 5.7, 5.8, 5.13, 7.1, 7.2, 7.3, 7.4 and 7.5.

August 1989   T. A. McNicholas

Contents

Contents

Contributors

S. G. Bown, MD, MRCP
Director, National Medical Laser Centre, Department of Surgery, University College Hospital, Gower Street, London WC1, UK

S. Flemming, MB BS, FRCS
Senior Registrar, Department of Plastic Surgery, Whiston Hospital, Whiston, Merseyside L35 5DR, UK
(Formerly Research Fellow, National Medical Laser Centre)

J. I. Harty, MD, LRCPSI, FRCSI, FACS
Assistant Professor, Department of Urology, Department of Surgery, University of Louisville, Louisville, Kentucky, USA
(Formerly Urological Research Fellow, National Medical Laser Centre)

H. B. Lottmann, MD
Chef de Clinique Urologique, Service d'Urologie, Hôpital Henri Mondor, 51 avenue du Maréchal de Lattre de Tassigny, 94000 Creteil, France
(Formerly Urological Research Fellow, National Medical Laser Centre)

T. A. McNicholas, MB BS, FRCS
Senior Registrar, St Peter's Group of Hospitals and The Middlesex Hospital, London WC2, UK

T. N. Mills, PhD
Senior Physicist, Department of Medical Physics, University College Hospital, Gower Street, London WC1, UK

R. O. Plail, BSc, MB BS, FRCS
Senior Registrar, Department of Urology, St Mary's Hospital, Praed Street, London W2, UK

A. J. Pope, BSc, MB BS, FRCS
Lecturer, Institute of Urology, 172 Shaftesbury Avenue, London WC2, UK

A. C. Steger, MB BS, FRCS
Research Fellow, Department of Surgery and National Medical
Laser Centre, University College Hospital, Gower Street, London
WC1, UK

G. M. Watson, MD, FRCS
Senior Lecturer, Institute of Urology and St Peter's Group of
Hospitals, 172 Shaftesbury Avenue, London WC2, UK

Chapter 1

An Introduction to Lasers and Laser Physics

T. N. Mills

This chapter offers an introduction to the laser and its principles of operation. Various laser types and the properties of laser light which make it suitable for medical use are also described.

Laser Physics

The Nature of Light

The word laser is an acronym for Light Amplification by Stimulated Emission of Radiation. To understand what is meant by this, it is first necessary to gain an understanding of the nature of light itself. It may be surprising to learn that light can take the form of both a particle and a wave. How science has arrived at and come to accept this duality will be described by taking a very brief and selective look at the history of optics.

The true nature of light has been the subject of conjecture and scientific investigation for many centuries. In the seventeenth century some researchers, including Sir Isaac Newton, favoured a corpuscular theory which treated light as being made up of a stream of particles or corpuscles. Others, of whom Robert Hooke and Christian Huygens were the principal proponents, preferred to consider light as being a wave propagating through an all-pervading elastic medium they called the "aether". Experimental evidence was available to support either theory. Fuelled by the considerable weight of Newton's opinion, yet contrary to his scientific philosophy, most scientists supported the corpuscular theory with tenacity and dogma, whilst the wave theory was all but stifled. Apart from a few notable exceptions, this state of affairs persisted until 1802, when Thomas Young and, a few years later, the Frenchman Jean Fresnel, revived the wave theory of light to explain the phenomena of diffraction, polarisation and interference. Young realised that light was a transverse wave, not a longitudinal wave; that is, the medium through which the wave propagated was disturbed in a direction perpendicular to rather than parallel with the direction of propagation.

The speed of light was first measured terrestrially by Armand Fizeau in 1849, and by the late nineteenth century was generally agreed to be about 300 000 km/s. Very importantly, its speed was found to be less in water than in air. Because Newton had predicted the reverse, this dealt what was thought to be the final blow to the corpuscular theory. The evidence now favoured the wave theory.

In 1867, James Clerk Maxwell, who had been analysing data of experiments on electricity and magnetism, particularly those of the arch-experimenter Michael Faraday, generated a set of equations which described exactly many of the observed properties of electricity and magnetism. An extraordinary result of this remarkable achievement was that the speed of propagation of a disturbance in an electromagnetic field, calculated using these equations, was exactly equal to the measured speed of light. Maxwell concluded that light was an electromagnetic wave whose propagation through the aether was determined solely by the electric and magnetic properties of the aether. The electromagnetic wave theory of light was met with utter disbelief until 8 years after Maxwell's death, when Heinrich Hertz discharged an induction coil across a spark gap to set up oscillating electric and magnetic fields and generate long-wavelength non-visible electromagnetic waves which could be reflected and refracted in exactly the same way as light.

So, light was an electromagnetic wave. But there remained a number of problems. Firstly, if it was assumed, as it had to be, that the earth and other celestial bodies moved relative to the stationary "aether", the speed of light measured in two different directions in space would be different. A famous experiment performed in 1887 by two Americans, Michelson and Morley, showed that this was not the case. The speed of light, which they were able to measure with very great accuracy, was the same in all directions. The problem was resolved in 1905, when Albert Einstein published his Special Theory of Relativity. He showed that electromagnetic waves were self-propagating: they had no need of the "aether", and the problems arising from its proposed existence could simply be forgotten.

The problems now remaining were concerned with the emission and absorption of light, which the wave theory was still unable to explain. For example, classical wave theory predicted that the intensity of radiation emitted by a "black body" should increase with decreasing wavelength. This would mean that as the wavelength decreased into the ultraviolet, the intensity of the radiation would become infinite. This "violet catastrophe" was not observed in practice. Max Planck, who treated the black body as being made up of numerous oscillating electric fields radiating electromagnetic waves, showed in 1900 that a satisfactory explanation could be obtained if the energies of the oscillators were restricted to only certain values.

Another puzzling phenomenon was observed by Hertz whilst studying the electrical discharge between two metal electrodes. He noticed that a spark was formed more readily when the electrodes were illuminated by ultraviolet light. Further studies revealed that the ultraviolet light prompted the release of electrons from the metallic surface of the cathode. Contrary to expectation, the effect did not disappear when the intensity of the light was reduced to below a particular level. Even at very low intensities, the effect persisted. Called the "photoelectric effect", this phenomenon could not be explained by the wave theory of light.

Building on the ideas originated by Max Planck, Einstein provided an explanation of the photoelectric effect. He treated light as being made up of discrete indivisible packets of energy, later to be called photons. The energy of each photon was inversely proportional to the wavelength of the light, such that ultraviolet light, which is of a short wavelength, is made up of photons having a high energy. Although the intensity of a beam of ultraviolet light may be very low, the energy of each photon was by itself sufficient to knock an electron off the metallic surface and reduce the voltage required to initiate a spark. It was for his explanation of the photoelectric effect, rather than his formulation of the Special and General Theories of Relativity, that Einstein was awarded the Nobel prize for physics in 1921.

The concept of the photon, whereby light takes the form of both a particle and a wave, formed the basis of an entirely new branch of physics dealing with the Quantum Theory of Matter. The quantum theory shows us that particle and wave are in fact different manifestations of the same thing, and, as stated by Einstein, that mass and energy are equivalent. The wavelength of radiation associated with a particle is inversely proportional to its momentum and so only sub-atomic particles, of which the photon is one, exhibit detectable wave-like properties.

Running apace with the studies on the nature of light, studies on the sub-microscopic world of the atom were also meeting with success. Fraunhofer at the beginning of the nineteenth century, as others before him, had noticed that the wavelengths of light emitted or absorbed by a particular element were confined to a number of narrow bands or spectral lines peculiar to that element. Rutherford a decade later had modelled the atom along the lines of our solar system, whereby the electrons orbited the atomic nucleus much as the planets orbit our sun. Whilst attractive in its simplicity, the model was flawed. Maxwell's laws, for example, suggested that the atom would radiate light continuously over a broad range of wavelengths, and the electrons would eventually collapse onto the nucleus.

In 1913, Neils Bohr used the newly formulated quantum theory to model the atom. The success of the new theory was demonstrated by its ability to predict accurately the wavelengths of the emission spectra of hydrogen. The emission and absorption of light could now be understood to result from changes in the energy of the atom, which the quantum theory shows to be restricted to certain defined values, each of which can be represented by a particular configuration of the extra-nuclear electrons. A change from one energy state to another is instantaneous and is accompanied by the absorption or emission of a packet of energy equal to the difference in energy between the two states, known as the transition energy. The packet of energy may be a photon of light. In molecules, other discrete energy levels are also present. These take the form of different stretching and rotational vibrations of the molecular bonds, and their transitions can also lead to photon emission.

The energy of the photon determines the wavelength of the electromagnetic radiation with which the photon is intrinsically associated. Thus a transition from one particular energy level to another produces radiation of just one wavelength. The greater the transition energy, the greater the photon energy and the shorter the wavelength, and vice versa. Light, which is taken to include the infrared, visible and ultraviolet, makes up only a small part of the

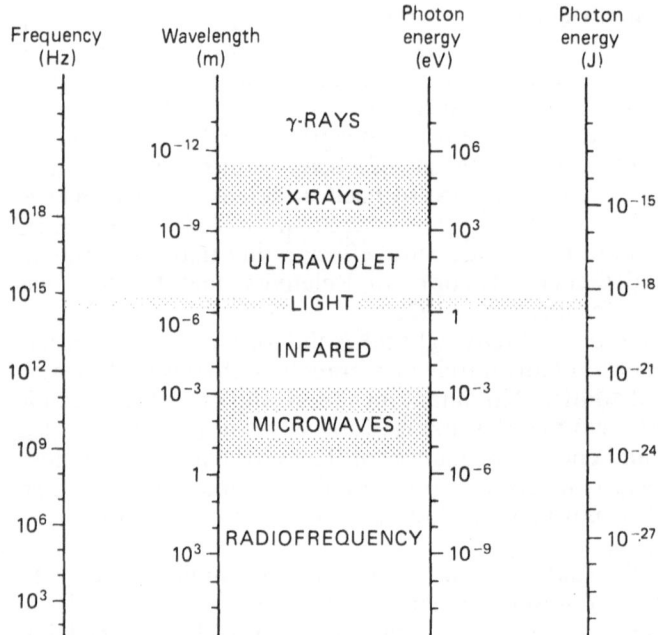

Fig. 1.1. The electromagnetic spectrum.

electromagnetic spectrum (see Fig. 1.1), the whole of which ranges from long-wavelength, low-frequency radio waves (low photon energy) to very-short-wavelength, very-high-frequency gamma rays (high photon energy).

Because the energy states of a particular species of atom are strictly defined, the transition and resultant photon energies are also strictly defined. An atom of one particular element, therefore, is able to absorb or emit photons of only particular energies, and hence only particular wavelengths. In actuality, the random movement of the atom and the close proximity of the external electric fields of adjacent atoms can increase or decrease the transition energies, resulting in emission of photons within a band of different energies, and hence wavelengths.

We have seen how our understanding of light has come more or less full circle. The emission and absorption of light are best considered using the photon and the quantum theory, similar in some respects to Newton's corpuscular theory, whilst the propagation of light is best considered using the classical electromagnetic wave theory. Together, the two theories provide a more or less complete description of the nature of light.

A Conventional Gas Discharge Light Source

Electric current flowing through the ionised gas in a gas discharge tube (e.g. a neon lamp) causes collisions which excite the atoms of the gas from the lowest-energy "ground state" to higher-energy "excited states". An atom excited to a high-energy state will in time return spontaneously to its low-energy ground state, either directly or via one or more intermediate states. Each transition is instantaneous and is accompanied by a release of energy equal to the difference in energy between the two states: the transition energy. The released transition energy may take the form of a photon of light. Photons released by these spontaneous radiative transitions are random in respect of phase, polarity and direction of propagation.

Atoms and molecules can exist only in certain strictly defined energy levels peculiar to their species. The transition and resultant photon energies are therefore also strictly defined. Thus, an atom of one particular element is able to absorb and emit photons of only certain energies, and hence only certain wavelengths. As stated earlier, the random movement of the atom and the close proximity of the external electric fields of adjacent atoms can affect the transition energies, resulting in emission of photons within a band of different energies, and hence wavelengths. The spectrum of light emitted by the gas discharge tube, therefore, is composed of one or more broad bands each spread about a central wavelength. Because the photons are emitted spontaneously, the light is emitted in all directions and with random phase and polarity.

Stimulated Emission and the Laser

Einstein, in 1917, showed that the relaxation of an excited atom or molecule to release a photon could happen not only spontaneously but also as a result of interaction with another photon of the correct energy. Remarkably, the incident photon remains unchanged and the newly emitted photon is identical to the incident photon in respect of wavelength, phase, polarisation and direction of propagation. The process is called "stimulated emission" and is the principle upon which laser action is based.

The practical significance of Einstein's discovery was not realised until after World War II, when it was found that conventional electronic devices were unable to amplify the very-high-frequency microwaves being used for radar. Nikolai Basov, Alexander Prokhorov and Charles H. Townes, amongst others, realised that a photon emitted by an excited atom or molecule could, by initiating a chain of repeated interactions with other excited atoms or molecules of the same species, stimulate the emission of numerous other identical photons. Thus, the intensity or flux of the electromagnetic wave associated with the original photon would be amplified. A prerequisite of this phenomenon was that there must be more atoms or molecules in the upper level, high-energy state than in the lower level, low-energy state, otherwise photons would tend to be absorbed by the lower level rather than stimulate emission of further photons from the upper level. Boltzmann's Law showed that this "population inversion" could not be obtained easily.

In 1953, Townes overcame the difficulties of obtaining a population inversion and constructed the first maser, an acronym for Microwave Amplification by Stimulated Emission of Radiation. Shortly thereafter, Townes and Arthur Schawlow set out the conditions necessary for Light Amplification by Stimulated Emission of Radiation: the laser.

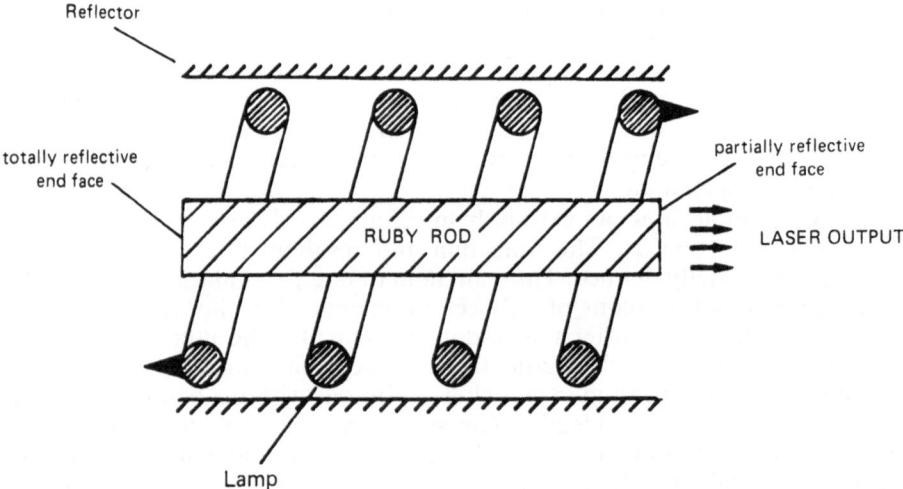

Fig. 1.2. The first laser.

The first laser, shown schematically in Fig. 1.2, was constructed by Theodore H. Maiman in 1960 whilst working at the Hughes Research Laboratory in the United States. To acknowledge this milestone in the history of optics, the Nobel prize for physics was awarded jointly to the American, Townes, and the two Russians, Basov and Prokhorov, in 1964.

The First Laser

As first suggested by Schawlow, Maiman used a small rod of synthetic ruby as the laser medium. Ruby is predominantly Al_2O_3 with a small percentage of Cr_3O_4 held in the crystal lattice. Its pale pink colour is attributable to absorption of light in the green and violet parts of the spectrum by the Cr^{3+} ions. It is a radiative transition of the excited ions on their path back to the ground state that is able to produce laser action.

Maiman polished the two end faces of the ruby rod flat and parallel, then silvered them such that light travelling parallel to the longitudinal axis would be reflected back and forth through the ruby rod. To allow some light to escape he left one face only partially silvered. The energy needed to excite the Cr^{3+} ions and produce the population inversion necessary for laser action was provided by a gas discharge flash lamp. Optical coupling between the flash lamp and the ruby was maximised by wrapping the lamp into a helix around the rod and enclosing the whole in a cylindrical reflector.

Fig. 1.3 shows a simplification of the energy levels in the ruby. Cr^{3+} ions are excited to high energy levels by the absorption of green and violet light emitted by the flash lamp. The absorption bands are very short lived and decay almost immediately to a metastable state via non-radiative transitions; the transition energy is lost as heat in the crystal lattice. The metastable state is relatively long lived and returns to the ground state via radiative transitions centred around 694 nm. Because the absorption bands decay very rapidly to a longer lived

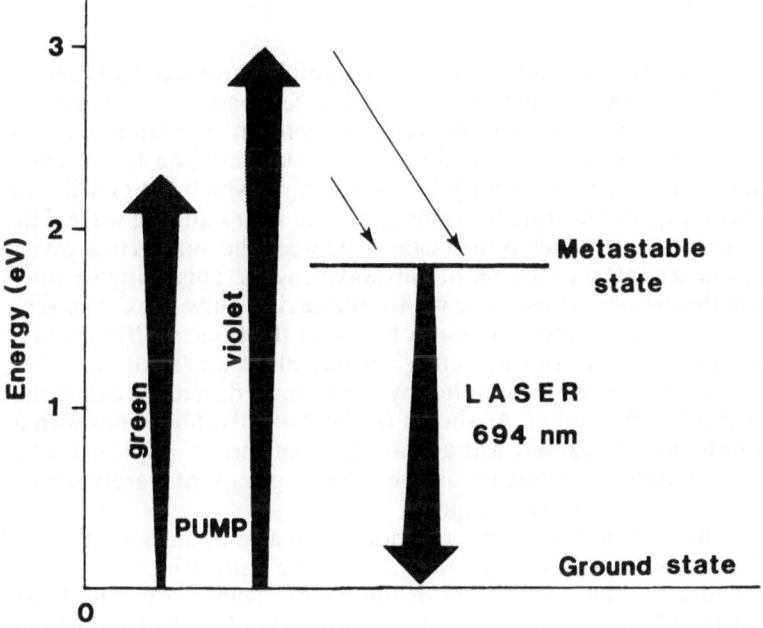

Fig. 1.3. Energy levels in ruby.

metastable state, a population inversion between metastable and ground states is readily achieved. Laser action is therefore possible.

Laser oscillation is initiated by a photon travelling in a direction parallel to the longitudinal axis of the rod and originating from the spontaneous relaxation of an excited Cr^{3+} ion. Along its path the photon interacts with another excited ion to stimulate the emission of a second, identical photon which propagates in the same direction. The two resultant photons stimulate the emission of yet more identical photons by further interactions with other excited ions. The chain reaction, of which these are the first steps, continues as the photons travel back and forth through the ruby rod, and lasts for almost as long as the population inversion remains. The result is an intense pulse of highly collimated red light emerging from the partially reflective end face of the rod.

Photons travelling in directions not parallel to the axis of the rod leak out through the side walls and are lost. They remove only a small amount of energy from the crystal. Some energy is lost within the crystal itself and at the two end mirrors; this does reduce the efficiency of the laser. The term "laser threshold" is used to describe the minimum population inversion needed to overcome the losses and initiate lasing.

Since Maiman's construction of the ruby laser, numerous other materials have been made to lase. These include gases, solids and liquids. To excite or pump the laser medium, electric currents, radio waves, light and even chemical reactions have been used. Unlike the first laser, some produce a continuous optical output, whilst others emit a series of extremely short, very powerful pulses.

Laser Cavity Modes

The laser is an oscillator, made up of an optical amplifier provided by the population inversion in the active medium, and optical feedback provided by the two end mirrors. Note that because the laser is more an oscillator than an amplifier, the acronym laser is something of a misnomer! The laser cavity takes the form of what is called a Fabry-Perot etalon, in which light oscillates between two plane-parallel mirrors forming, as it does so, a standing wave. The length of the standing wave, which is the distance between the mirrors (the cavity length), must equal an integer number of half wavelengths. This being so, only certain wavelengths are able to oscillate within the cavity. Thus, the cavity separates each of the broad radiative emission bands of the laser medium into a number of very narrow bands or lines, each attributable to an "axial mode" of the cavity, and separated from one another by a frequency difference called the "free spectral range" of the etalon. As shown in Fig. 1.4, only those lines with a gain exceeding the laser threshold will actually lase and so be amplified. The output of a laser, therefore, is made up of one or more groups of closely separated narrow lines or bands of wavelengths.

In addition to the axial mode, transverse modes can also be sustained in the laser cavity. These describe light which resonates along paths which do not lie exactly parallel to the longitudinal axis of the cavity. They are called TEM (Transverse Electro-Magnetic) modes, and are designated by TEM-mn where m and n denote the number of transverse nodal lines appearing across the output beam along the horizontal and vertical axes respectively. In other words, the output beam may be split up into one or more regions. A variety of different

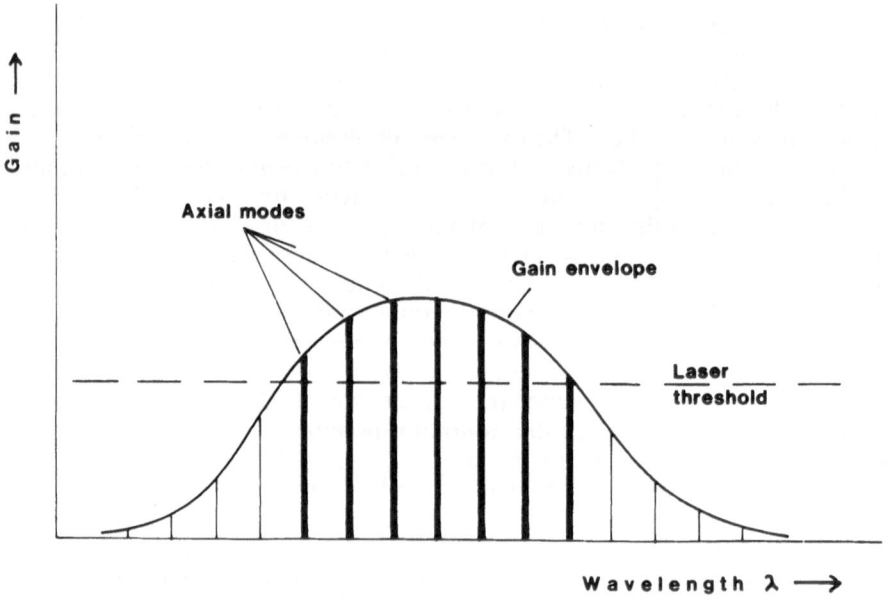

Fig. 1.4. Gain curve of a laser emission showing the axial modes of the laser cavity.

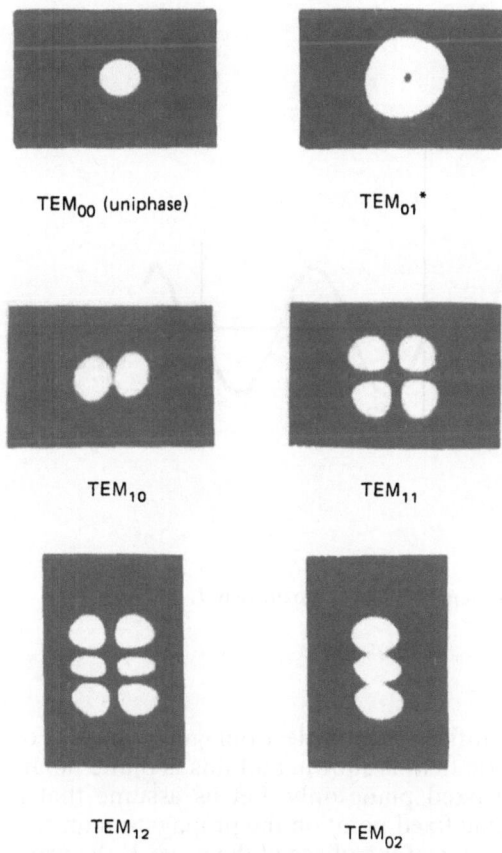

Fig. 1.5. Some low-order transverse electric and magnetic (TEM) modes of a laser.

modes are shown in Fig. 1.5. For a number of reasons the lowest-order mode, TEM-00, is the most widely used: not only is the distribution of flux density or irradiance (power per unit area) across the beam ideally Gaussian, but the electric field exhibits no phase changes, which means it is completely "spatially coherent", it exhibits the least beam divergence, and it can be focused to the smallest spot size.

Coherence

Light is energy propagating through space as an electromagnetic wave. We can characterise light by the wavelength and amplitude of the electromagnetic wave. Furthermore, we can say how stable the wave is with respect to both time and position in space. These last two observations describe the temporal coherence and spatial coherence of the light.

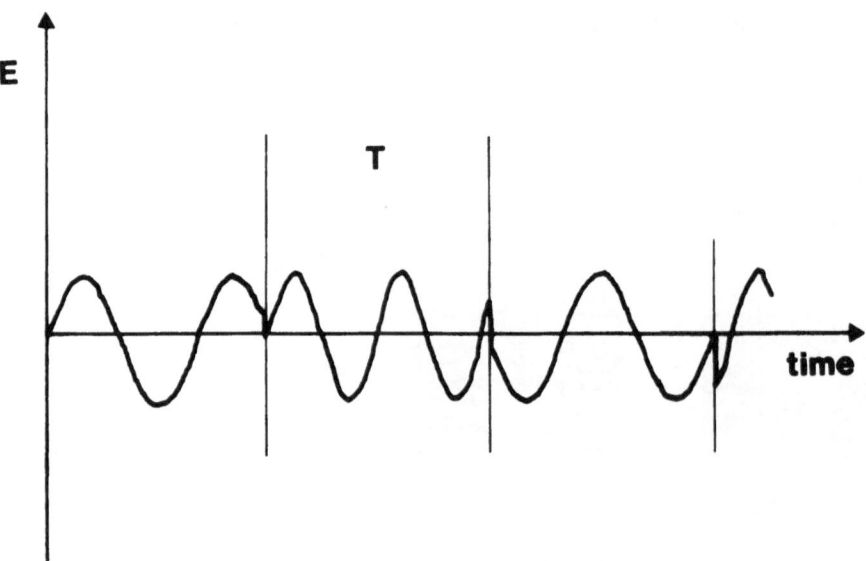

Fig. 1.6. An electromagnetic wave with a coherence time of approximately *T*.

Temporal Coherence

Fig. 1.6 depicts a short length of an infinitely long electromagnetic wave. For the sake of simplicity, only the electric field is shown, and this is plane polarised, i.e. the field oscillates in one fixed plane only. Let us assume that a stationary observer, positioned at some fixed point on the propagation axis, is able to take instantaneous measurements of the phase of the wave. If the wave is of just one frequency (and thus of one wavelength), the observer will know the relationship between the phase of the wave at the instant of measurement and the phase at any later instant. If, however, the frequency of the wave is subject to change, the phase relationship will only hold for as long as the frequency remains constant. This is called the "coherence time". The same property can be described equally well by the length of the wave over which the frequency remains constant. This is called the "coherence length", and is, of course, equal to the product of the speed of light and the coherence time. Either quantity serves to describe the temporal coherence of the light.

The wavelength distribution, or spectral linewidth, of light is also a measure of its temporal coherence, and is related to the coherence time (or coherence length). The natural linewidth, which is the linewidth of the spectral emission of a single stationary atom, is greatly broadened by heat and the presence of other atoms. This is due to distribution of the atomic energy levels caused by collisions, thermal oscillations, and the close proximity of the external electric fields of the other atoms. Due in part to the process of stimulated emission, and in part to the geometry of the laser cavity, the spectral linewidth of the output of a laser is very much narrower than that of a conventional light source.

Coherence lengths of many hundreds of kilometres are possible from a laser, but few commercially available lasers have coherence lengths of more than a

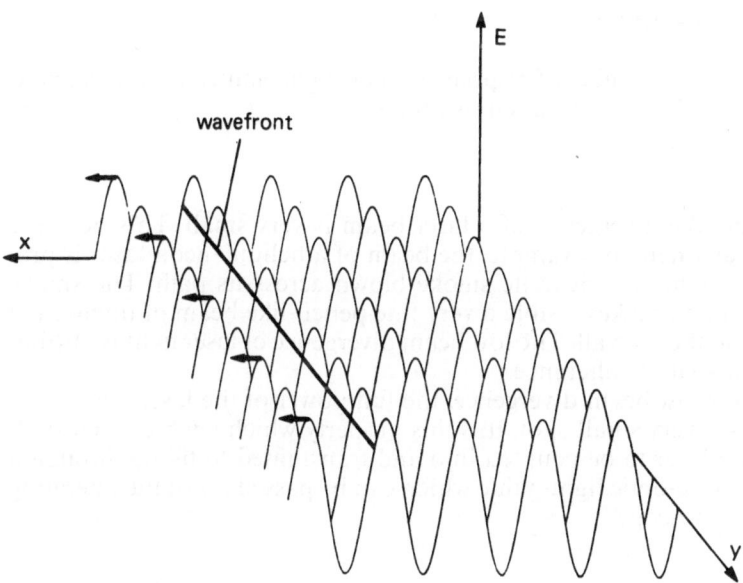

Fig. 1.7. A perfectly collimated, spatially coherent beam of light. The wavefront is drawn through two points of equal phase.

few tens of metres. This implies coherence times of less than 1 microsecond. Conventional light sources have coherence lengths of less than 1 mm.

Spatial Coherence

Spatial coherence is concerned with the stability of the relative phases of a wave at two points in space – rather than two points in time, as in the case with temporal coherence. To see what is meant by this, we need to refer to Fig. 1.7, which shows a number of wavetrains of a perfectly collimated beam of light. A wavefront, which is depicted by the bold line, is drawn through points on the wavetrains that have equal phase. Spatial coherence implies that all wavefronts which arrive subsequently at this same position in space will have the same shape. The wavetrains may change frequency because of the relative brevity of the coherence time, but, provided the wavefronts maintain the same shape, the light is spatially coherent.

The wavefront of a spatially coherent point source is a spherical shell centred on the source. Similarly, a perfectly collimated beam of light infers a flat wavefront and perfect spatial coherence.

In summary, temporal coherence implies that the relative phases between two points in time remain constant; spatial coherence, on the other hand, implies that the relative phases between two points in space remain constant.

It should be noted that a conventional light source can produce coherent light, but only in passing it through narrow slits and a filter, after which the power of the beam is too low to be of any real value. Only the laser is able to produce powerful temporally and spatially coherent light.

Properties of Laser Light

Laser light differs in a number of respects from the light emitted by, for example, a domestic light bulb or a gas discharge tube.

Beam Collimation

By any criterion, the divergence of a laser beam is very small. This becomes abundantly clear when, for example, the beam of a helium–neon laser is projected across a room and cigarette smoke blown across its path. The smoke scatters the light and makes visible a very fine pencil-like beam of intense red light stretching to the far wall. The low beam divergence of laser light is attributable to its high spatial coherence.

Because of this low beam divergence, the full power of the laser beam may be focused onto a very small spot. It is this property which enables almost all the power of the laser to be coupled into and transmitted to tissue through a small-diameter fibre-optic light-guide which can be passed down the operating channel of an endoscope.

Output Power

An important consequence of the high collimation of a laser beam is that although the power output of the laser may be less than that of, say, a fluorescent lamp, the irradiance (power per unit cross-sectional area) of the beam is very high and can remain so for up to very great distances. In contrast a fluorescent lamp emits light in all directions as an approximately spherical wave the irradiance of which decreases as the inverse square of the distance from the lamp. It is almost impossible to arrange a conventional light source to produce a collimated beam of light with an irradiance comparable to that of a laser.

A further consequence of the low divergence of the laser beam is that it may be focused onto a very small spot to produce still greater irradiance. The minimum diameter of the focused beam is a function of the angle of divergence of the laser and the focal length of the lens. The ultimate spot size is determined by the wavelength of light, i.e. the spot is "diffraction limited". Spot diameters of the order of only a few hundredths of a millimetre can be readily obtained. The consequent irradiance may be some million million times that attained in an oxyacetylene flame.

Monochromaticity

Laser light is monochromatic or, more precisely, quasi-monochromatic. It is light of just one or a few colours. The output of a laser, therefore, is a beam of light the entire output power of which may be centred on more or less one wavelength. With a conventional light source, the light is found to be spread over a very much broader band of wavelengths. The monochromaticity of laser light is attributable to its high temporal coherence.

Most laser media possess a number of radiative emission bands which are able to lase, each attributable to particular transitions within the atom or molecule. The output, therefore, may consist of light of a number of different colours. The argon laser, for example, can lase at about eleven different wavelengths between 437 nm and 529 nm. If only one particular wavelength is required, output at the unwanted wavelengths may be prevented by a variety of techniques. Most often, the back (totally reflecting) mirror is a multilayered dielectric stack such that unwanted wavelengths are attenuated by destructive interference occurring at each multiple reflection within the mirror. Other techniques make use of prisms or diffraction gratings.

Polarisation of Light

Some lasers, by the nature of their construction, emit plane polarised light, that is, the electric field of the light oscillates in only one plane perpendicular to the direction of propagation. There is, as yet, little evidence to substantiate claims that the polarisation of light plays a part in its interaction with tissue.

Interaction of Laser Light with Tissue

When light enters tissue, it is scattered and absorbed. The phenomenon of scattering is exemplified by light propagating through fog: the light is bounced back and forth between water droplets, spreading the light out in all directions. Absorption, on the other hand, is where the light is captured by the medium, which may then convert its energy into heat.

The practical, clinical importance of the monochromaticity of laser light is that one component of tissue may absorb or scatter light of one wavelength more strongly than another. The blue-green light of the argon ion laser, for example, is strongly absorbed by red blood, but relatively weakly absorbed by dermis and epidermis. The absorbed light energy is converted to heat, and so, when skin is irradiated with argon laser light, the temperature of the capillary blood may be raised to a higher temperature than is the dermis or the epidermis. The abnormal blood-filled capillaries of a port wine stain may therefore be destroyed with minimal damage to the skin. The selectivity of this effect is maximised if the light energy is delivered using a pulsed laser in which the duration of the pulses is shorter than the time it takes heat to diffuse out of the capillaries and into the surrounding dermis. The time the laser is switched off, between individual pulses is also important. It needs to be longer than this characteristic "thermal diffusion time", otherwise individual pulses summate to have the effect of a single, longer pulse. The thermal diffusion time of a capillary blood vessel within the dermis is of the order of 1 millisecond.

In liver, blue-green argon laser light penetrates to a depth of about 1 mm. The invisible near-infrared light of the neodymium yttrium aluminium garnet (YAG) laser, which is less strongly absorbed by liver, penetrates to a depth of about 5 mm, and, because of scattering, is spread sideways away from the axis of the incident beam. The longer wavelength far-infrared light of the carbon dioxide (CO_2) laser, which is absorbed very strongly by water, penetrates to a depth of only about 0.1 mm in liver. Because the degree of absorption and scattering determines the volume of tissue in which the light energy is dissipated, the power density in tissue irradiated by a CO_2 laser may be sufficiently high to cause explosive vaporisation of intracellular water. This phenomenon forms the basis of the use of the CO_2 laser as a tissue cutter or "laser scalpel". The more deeply penetrating but more powerful YAG laser heats a greater volume of tissue more gradually, which is ideal for coagulation.

Light can produce a number of non-thermal effects in tissue. It can activate photochemical reactions in much the same way that sunlight absorbed by chlorophyll activates photosynthesis. Alternatively, if the light is of a short wavelength (e.g. ultraviolet light), the photon energies may be sufficiently high to disrupt directly the molecular bonds within tissue. The latter effect, called photoablation, might form the basis of a "cold" laser scalpel.

At very high power densities, such as those attainable in the very short duration pulses produced by a Q-switched laser, the electric field strengths are high enough to disrupt the atomic structure of tissue. Electrons are torn from atomic nuclei to form a very hot but very localised plasma. By focusing Q-switched laser pulses through the ocular lens and onto the posterior capsule, ophthalmologists can use this effect to perform posterior capsulotomies without resort to surgery. With the recent development of a suitable fibre-optic delivery system, the Q-switched laser can also be used to generate destructive shock waves for the fragmentation of urinary and biliary calculi. The shock waves are produced by the rapidly expanding plasma formed at the point of impact of the Q-switched laser pulse.

Clinical Lasers and Laser Light Delivery

This section offers a brief description of each of the laser types which have proved to be or promise to be of particular value in urology.

Argon Ion Laser

The laser medium of the argon ion laser is a volume of argon gas held in a small-diameter, air or water cooled tube made of glass, graphite or beryllium oxide and sealed at each end by glass windows. A current, constricted by a magnetic field and flowing between electrodes positioned within each end of the tube, ionises the argon gas and excites the ions so formed to high-energy states. Transitions between high-energy absorption states and a lower-energy intermediate state release photons of light in the blue-green part of the spectrum. Mirrors positioned outside each end of the tube reflect the photons back and forth through the gas. At very high current densities, a population inversion between absorption states and the intermediate state exists, stimulated emission predominates over absorption, and laser oscillation occurs. To minimise losses, the windows at each end of the tube are tilted at the "Brewster angle". This is the angle at which light polarised in the plane normal to the window is transmitted with maximum efficiency.

One of the two mirrors, the output mirror, is only partially silvered. The laser output which emerges from this mirror is a highly collimated beam of plane polarised light made up of a number of different spectral lines or wavelengths lying between 437 nm and 529 nm (80% of the power is equally divided between 488 nm and 514.5 nm). There are also a number of less powerful lines which can lase in the ultraviolet part of the spectrum.

The full output power of the argon ion laser suitable for medical use can be readily coupled into an optical fibre sufficiently small and flexible to be passed down the operating channel of a standard flexible endoscope. Like the majority of lasers, the argon ion laser is very inefficient. An 8-W device, for example, requires an electrical input power of about 15 kW. This usually necessitates a three-phase electrical service and a substantial supply of cooling water.

Neodymium Yttrium Aluminium Garnet Laser

The laser medium of the neodymium yttrium aluminium garnet laser is a synthetic crystal rod of yttrium aluminium garnet (YAG) which has been doped with a small concentration of neodymium (Nd) atoms. Light emitted by a powerful krypton lamp, and focused into the rod by an elliptical reflector, "pumps" the neodymium atoms into a broad band of high-energy states which rapidly decay via non-radiative transitions to long-lived metastable states. Lasing, predominantly at the near-infrared wavelength of 1064 nm, results from the decay of these metastable states to lower-energy intermediate states, which then decay rapidly via non-radiative transitions to the ground state. Called a four-level laser, a population inversion and consequent lasing is readily achieved between the long-lived, high-energy states and the short-lived, low-energy intermediate states. The laser cavity is completed by mirrors positioned at each end of the rod. One mirror, the output mirror, is only partially silvered, whilst the other is usually multicoated to allow only the desired wavelength to lase.

The efficiency of the YAG laser is relatively high at between 1% and 2%. Continuous wave output powers in excess of 1 kW are possible, but for clinical applications, 100 W at 1064 nm is ample. Despite its relatively high efficiency, a YAG laser of this power requires a three-phase electrical service and a supply of cooling water. To enable visualisation of the path of the invisible infrared beam, a coaxial visible red beam of a low-power helium–neon laser is usually employed. Both visible red and near-infrared beams can be transmitted by small-diameter optical fibres.

Carbon Dioxide Laser

Lying deep in the infrared at 10.6 μm the output beam of the carbon dioxide (CO_2) laser is absorbed strongly by all conventional optical fibres. Whilst this precludes its present use with flexible endoscopes, it is likely that a suitable fibre will be made available in the near future.

The laser medium of the CO_2 laser is a mixture of carbon dioxide, nitrogen and helium gas, held in an air or water cooled discharge tube sealed at each end by Brewster windows transparent to the infrared. Lasing occurs at transitions between quantised vibrational states of the carbon dioxide molecule, excited by energy transferred from the nitrogen molecules which are themselves excited by direct or alternating currents. The presence of helium helps provide the population inversion by cooling the lower lasing level of the CO_2 molecule to its ground state. The resonant cavity is, as usual, provided by two mirrors positioned outside each end of the tube.

In comparison with other lasers, the CO_2 laser is very efficient, 15% efficiency being typical. Continuous wave output powers of a few kilowatts are attainable by some designs, but for most clinical uses a maximum of 35 W is ample. Because of its high efficiency, such a device can be powered by a single-phase electrical service and has no need of an external supply of cooling water. As with the YAG laser, a helium–neon laser provides a visible red aiming beam.

Dye Lasers

A laser ideal for clinical use would be a device with a high maximum output power and a wavelength tunable from infrared to the ultraviolet. Whilst not satisfying the former requirement, the dye laser goes a long way towards satisfying the latter.

The laser medium of the dye laser is a dye, such as a coumarin or rhodamine, in a solvent, such as ethanol. When liquid dye is excited by light of a short wavelength, transitions between the first excited electronic state and numerous vibrational levels of the ground state radiate (fluoresce) light within a broad band, about 70 nm wide. Different dyes lase within different ranges.

A tunable, continuous wave dye laser, just one of many different designs, is shown in Fig. 1.8. Liquid dye is pumped through a nozzle to form a thin, laminar jet which is directed across the optical path of a "folded, three mirror cavity". The liquid dye is then recirculated. At the point where the jet crosses the optical path of the cavity, the dye molecules are excited to a high-energy state by an intense beam of light, in this case originating from a continuous wave ion laser. At intensities greater than 1 MW/cm^2, population inversions between the first excited electronic state and the numerous vibrational levels of the ground state exist, and their transitions provide laser action at wavelengths within the fluorescence spectrum of the dye.

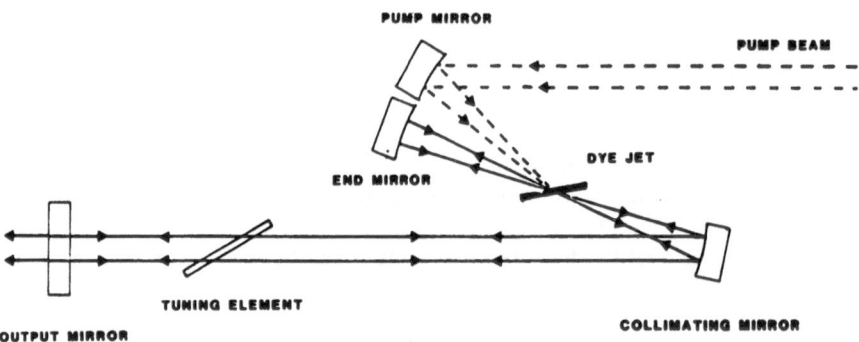

Fig. 1.8. A continuous-wave, tunable dye laser using a folded, three-mirror cavity and pumped by a continuous wave ion laser.

The high-velocity liquid jet restricts the flight time of the dye molecules through the active area to less than a microsecond. This is long compared with the fluorescence process, but is short compared with other processes such as phosphorescence which would tend to reduce the dye laser's efficiency. The birefringent crystal provides a means of tuning the wavelength of the laser output, i.e. for any one rotational position, light of only one wavelength can oscillate within the laser cavity.

The efficiency of the dye laser is high, reaching a maximum of about 25%. The efficiency of the complete system, however, is compromised by the low efficiency of the pump laser. Using a range of different dyes and optical cavity mirrors, a dye laser pumped by a 7-W continuous wave argon ion laser can lase at any wavelength between 430 nm and 900 nm, with a peak continuous wave output power of about 1.5 W.

In another design of dye laser, a flash lamp pumps the liquid dye to produce 1-microsecond pulses of typically 200 mJ per pulse. These pulses, which may be transmitted using flexible, small-diameter optical fibres, are effective for fragmenting urinary calculi and calcified arterial plaques.

Metal Vapour Lasers

A number of metals can be made to lase when in their vapour phase. They include copper, which lases at 511 nm (green) and 578 nm (yellow), and gold, which lases at 628 nm (red). The construction of a metal vapour laser follows the general scheme of a gas laser, but to obtain the required vapour densities the laser must operate at high temperatures. The laser tube is therefore usually made of alumina and the central portion may be held in an oven.

Described as self-terminating, metal vapour lasers can only operate in pulsed mode and (because they exhibit a very high gain per pass,) they are able to lase without any mirrors. To obtain a unidirectional output, however, a 100% reflecting mirror is positioned at one end of the laser tube and the output is taken directly from the other. The output specification of an air-cooled copper vapour laser is typically 1 mJ per pulse, 10 kHz pulse repetition frequency, 10 W average power.

Excimer Lasers

Excimer lasers are of great interest because they provide a source of ultraviolet laser light. The laser medium of an excimer laser is a volume of gas the atoms of which are able to form diatomic molecules only in an excited state. The molecules immediately dissociate, releasing high-energy ultraviolet photons on entering the ground state. A population inversion between excited and ground states and consequent laser action at ultraviolet wavelengths is therefore possible.

The word "excimer" is a contraction of the words "excited dimer", but often the active molecule is a rare gas atom combined in the excited state with a halogen atom. Strictly speaking these combinations should not be called excimers since they involve dissimilar atoms.

Specific examples of rare gas/halide excimer lasers are argon fluoride (193 nm), krypton fluoride (248 nm), xenon chloride (308 nm) and xenon fluoride

(351 nm). They may be pumped either by an electron beam or by an electrical discharge. The output is pulsed, the length of each pulse being of the order of a few tens of nanoseconds.

Q-Switched YAG Laser

In a conventional laser, laser oscillation begins as soon as the laser medium has been pumped to laser threshold. Preventing oscillation by means of a shutter placed within the laser cavity, the laser medium in a Q-switched laser can be pumped to a level far greater than threshold. When the shutter is eventually opened, the energy stored within the laser medium is released as a single optical pulse having a duration of about 10 nanoseconds. The peak power of such a pulse can be of the order of a gigawatt (10^9 W).

Fibre-optics

Total Internal Reflection

In the way copper cables are used to conduct electricity, optical fibres are used to transmit light. Optical fibres of the "step index" variety transmit light using the principle of total internal reflection. When a ray of light travelling in a medium of high refractive index meets another medium of lower refractive

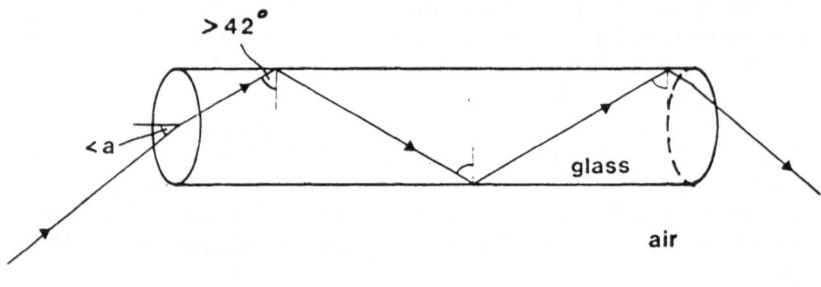

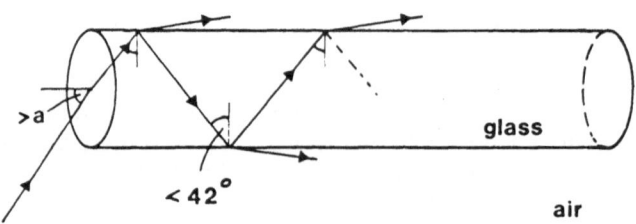

Fig. 1.9. Total internal reflection of light within a glass cylinder (refractive index = 1.5) surrounded by air (refractive index = 1). The critical angle of reflection at the glass/air boundary is 42°. The angle *a* is the acceptance angle of the cylinder.

index, the ray is reflected back into the first medium if its angle of incidence at the boundary is greater than the critical angle. The critical angle K is derived from the relationship

$$\sin K = n_2/n_1$$

where n_1 and n_2 are the refractive indices of the two media.

Fig. 1.9 shows a ray of light travelling in a solid cylinder of glass ($n = 1.5$) held in air ($n = 1$). On meeting the side wall of the cylinder, the ray is totally internally reflected if its angle of incidence is greater than 42°. Rays of light incident at angles of less than 42° leak out of the cylinder and into the air. It is easy to see that the glass cylinder can, by multiple total internal reflections, transmit light along its full length, provided the light starts its journey running in a direction lying close to the longitudinal axis of the cylinder, i.e. within the "acceptance angle", a.

Commercially available step index optical fibres are made up of a cylindrical core of glass or fused silica which is isolated from the external environment by a layer of lower refractive index glass or polymer, called the cladding. The whole may be then enclosed in a tough plastic sheath for protection. The cladding, by providing an optically smooth boundary at the wall of the fibre core, minimises transmission losses.

Low loss fibres are available commercially in sizes ranging from about 10 μm to 1000 μm in diameter. Fibres made of glass are suitable for transmitting light in the 380–1300 nm range, whilst those made of fused silica are suitable for wavelengths of 220–1300 nm. Flexible fibre-optic endoscopes utilise bundles of the smaller-diameter glass fibres for both illumination and image transmission. For transmitting laser light down the biopsy channel of an endoscope, single fibres of larger diameter are employed.

In addition to the step index fibres, there is also a family of "graded index" fibres. Although graded index fibres are not normally used for transmitting high-power laser light, the way in which they work may be of some interest. The refractive index of the cores of graded index fibres varies continuously with radius, from a high value at the centre to a low value at the surface. The cladding is absent. Rays of light not travelling parallel to the axis of the fibre are deflected by refraction away from the surface and back towards the centre. The fibre acts rather like a series of positive lenses, each re-imaging the image formed by the previous lens. In many respects these fibres are similar to the rod lenses used in rigid urological endoscopes.

Fibre-optic Transmission of Laser Light

The property of the laser which enables its use in therapeutic endoscopy is the very low divergence of its output beam. It allows almost all the energy of the laser to be coupled into and transmitted by an optical fibre sufficiently small and flexible to be passed down the biopsy channel of a standard endoscope. The smallest spot to which a laser beam can be focused is calculated using the relationship

$$d = 2f \sin A$$

where d is the spot diameter, f the focal length of the coupling lens, and A the angle of divergence of the laser.

To ensure efficient transmission of the laser energy by an optical fibre, the angle of convergence of the focused beam must not, of course, exceed the acceptance angle of the fibre.

Whilst the output beam of a YAG laser can be focused to a spot diameter of about 200 μm, an optical fibre of about 400 μm diameter is usually employed for use with an endoscope. The larger diameter facilitates accurate alignment, which ensures efficient coupling of the laser energy into the fibre.

To minimise power loss, the two ends of the fibre must be cleaved flat and perpendicular to the longitudinal axis. They must be clean; any dirt will absorb energy, get hot, and melt the fibre tip. The risk of contamination can be reduced by providing a coaxial gas jet.

The laser light emerges from the distal end of the fibre as a divergent cone. The irradiance at the tissue surface is therefore dependent upon the cone angle and the fibre tip to tissue separation.

Optical Fibres for the CO_2 Laser

The light emitted by the CO_2 laser lies deep in the infrared region of the electromagnetic spectrum. Light of this wavelength (10.6 μm) is absorbed very strongly by many materials, including those used in conventional optical fibres. Most of the materials which do not absorb 10.6 μm light have either poor mechanical properties or high toxicity, both of which render them unsuitable as optical fibres for clinical use. At the time of writing, considerable effort is being devoted to the development of an endoscopic "CO_2 fibre"; this will, no doubt, soon bear fruit.

Laser Safety

Lasers are hazardous. Their clinical use is associated with a number of potential hazards to the patient, operator and staff. Their use requires extreme caution.

The eye is at greatest risk. The ocular lens, like any other positive lens, focuses the highly collimated beam of the laser to a very small spot. In the eye, this spot falls on the retina. Because the full power of the laser beam is concentrated within the area of this spot, part of the retina may be instantly and permanently destroyed if the power of the laser beam entering the eye exceeds a certain critical value. Almost all clinical lasers mentioned in this chapter exceed this critical value by at least three orders of magnitude. The exceptions cannot damage the retina by virtue of the fact that their beams are absorbed very strongly by water, resulting in corneal burns and permanent scarring rather than retinal damage.

If there is any possibility of the laser beam entering the eye, either directly or by reflection, and exceeding the maximum permissible exposure level, protective eyewear which attenuates the laser beam to a safe level must be worn. Of particular relevance to the use of lasers with endoscopes is the provision of a filter or shutter at the eyepiece of the endoscope. This prevents reflected light from entering the operator's eye via the optics of the endoscope.

Apart from the risk of damage to the eye, the laser presents a fire hazard and can produce serious burns to exposed skin.

All personnel associated with the use of clinical lasers should read the manufacturer's operating instructions, be aware of the hazards and take all necessary steps to minimise the risk of accidents. A number of publications devoted entirely to the subject of laser safety are listed in Further Reading.

Further Reading

Optics

Barton AW (1939) A textbook on light. Longman, Harlow
Fowles GR (1968) Introduction to modern optics. Holt, Rinehart and Winston, New York
Goldwasser EL (1965) Optics, waves, atoms and nuclei: an introduction. Benjamin, New York
Hecht E, Zajac A (1982) Optics. Addison-Wesley, Reading, Mass.
Jenkins FA, White HE (1957) Fundamentals of optics. McGraw-Hill, New York
Van Heel ACS, Velzel CHF (1968) What is light? McGraw-Hill, New York

Lasers

Beasley MJ (1978) Lasers and their applications. Taylor and Francis, London
Carruth JAS, McKenzie A (1986) Medical lasers. Adam Hilger, Bristol
Heavens OS (1971) Lasers. Duckworth, London
Lengyl BA (1962) Lasers: generation of light by stimulated emission. Wiley, New York
Schawlow AL (1969) Lasers and light: readings from *Scientific American*. Freeman, Oxford
Svelto O (1982) Principles of lasers. Plenum Press, New York
Thyagarajan K, Ghatak AK (1981) Lasers: theory and applications. Plenum Press, New York

Fibre-optics

Cherin AH (1983) Introduction to optical fibres. McGraw-Hill, New York
Okoshi T (1982) Optical fibres. Academic Press, New York London
Wolf HF (ed) (1979) Handbook of fibre optics. Granada, London

Safety

BSI (1983) BS 4803: radiation safety of laser products and systems. Parts 1, 2 and 3. British Standards Institution, London
HMSO (1985) Guidance on the safe use of lasers in medical practice. Her Majesty's Stationery Office, London
Lerman S (1980) Radiant energy and the eye. Macmillan, London
Mallow A, Chabot L (1978) Laser safety handbook. Van Nostrand Reinhold, New York
Sliney DH, Wolbarsht ML (1980) Safety with lasers and other optical sources. Plenum Press, New York

Chapter 2

A Practical Guide to Laser Treatment

T. A. McNicholas

This chapter sets out general guidance for laser use with special reference to the endoscopic YAG coagulation of bladder tumours, since these are of general importance to all urologists. The practical points outlined here will have relevance to most other urological laser applications. Where particular points are important for specific applications they will be dealt with in the appropriate chapters later in the book. Table 2.1 describes the characteristics of lasers in urological use.

General Guidance

A close liaison between the urologist and the manufacturer of the laser he eventually chooses is essential. Time and effort spent assessing the various machines is time well spent. In effect this means reading the literature and

Table 2.1. Characteristics of lasers in urological use

Laser	Wavelength (nm)	Power range (W)	Mode	Delivery system	Use
CO_2	10 600	0.1–100	CW[a] + pulsed	Articulated arm to endoscope or microscope	Cutting, tissue welding
Argon	458–515	0.001–25	CW + pulsed	Fibre	Superficial coagulation
Dye	400–700	0.001–6	CW + pulsed	Fibre.	Photodynamic therapy (PDT), laser lithotripsy
YAG	1060	5–120	CW + pulsed Q-switched	Fibre	Coagulation (tumours and vascular lesions)

[a]CW, continuous wave.

then talking to other users and subsequently meeting the manufacturers and assessing their products. We would suggest that although a great deal of information can be gained from the literature and colleagues it is essential to see at least the "short listed" machines in operation in the environment in which you plan to use them. This may require some temporary safety measures for the purpose of the short trial period, but do not make expensive alterations prior to purchase of the laser. A practical trial in your own operating room will show whether the laser can work with existing electrical and water supplies. However, the hospital engineers can usually advise about the electrical supply and water temperatures and flow rates which are available. Ideally, expensive alterations such as water pumps or cooling arrangements for the water (if the ambient temperature is high) should be avoided. Fig. 2.1. shows our clinical laser installed in the operating theatre at St. Peter's Hospital, London.

We cannot stress strongly enough how important a good relationship between the operator and the manufacturer is. Good back-up service is perhaps the single most important feature to look for, though the current range of lasers themselves (particularly YAG and CO_2 lasers) are really quite reliable instruments.

After buying the laser local safety rules may have to be drawn up or may already be in existence due to laser use in other departments. We would advise a period of training with an experienced laser operator if there is one practising nearby, although there are many "hands-on" courses available. These should allow some practical guidance on the use of the laser and practical experience on dead tissue, subsequently on live tissue and possibly demonstration of clinical cases.

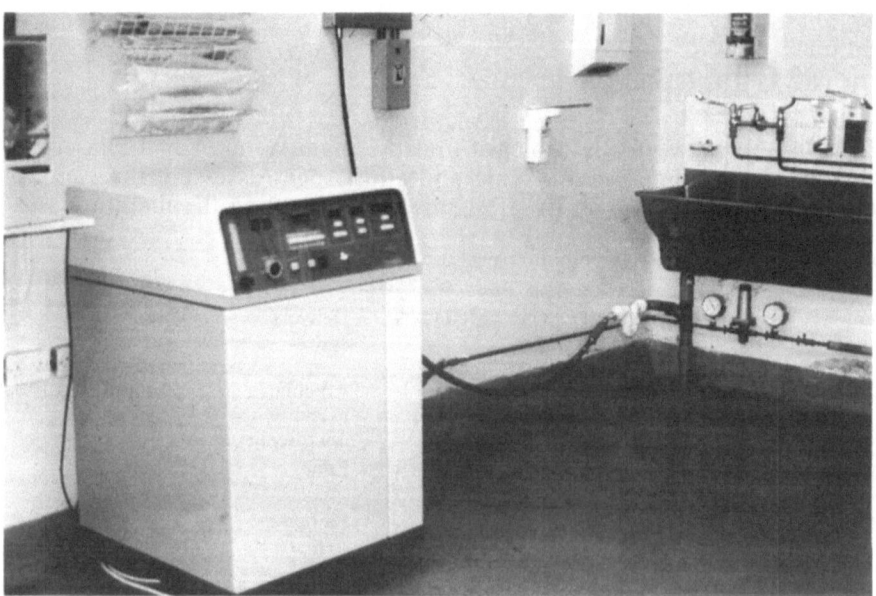

Fig. 2.1. The Living Technology Fiberlase in the operating theatre at St. Peter's Hospital, London. (Reproduced by permission of the *British Journal of Hospital Medicine.*)

The laser operator should be aware that in British practice he is likely to be the one who has, in the final analysis, to make the machine work, although in more affluent environments elsewhere the resources may be available for a laser technician or perhaps a nurse dedicated to looking after the laser. In either case at least one person should be intimately familiar with the standard operation of the laser and be able to deal with simple malfunctions. For more serious problems a "hot line" to the manufacturers or their agents is essential and that 'phone number should be available to the user at all times.

The choice of laser is at least partly determined by price. Machines of increasing sophistication are becoming available, but unfortunately usually at an increased price. However, some recent technological developments are worthy of further consideration. The advent of YAG lasers that can function reliably without requiring a continuous supply of running water and which can draw their power requirements from relatively routine electrical circuits would be a great advantage for many people. Savings in the cost of electrical and plumbing alterations and fittings might well outweigh some of the extra cost of the new machines. These new developments also mean that the machines are more mobile and can more easily be moved from one operating room to another.

Purchase and installation of the laser in an appropriate operating room having been successfully completed, the urologist has to choose appropriate cases for treatment. We would advise gaining experience on simple superficial bladder cancers and some skin lesions such as viral warts of the genitalia which will allow use of the "non-urological fibres" that generally require cooling with gas (Figs. 2.2 and 2.3).

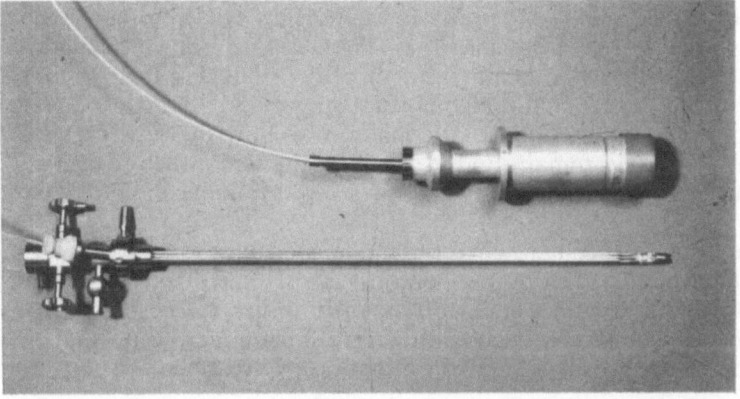

Fig. 2.2. A fibre delivery system (urological system: bare fibre with PTFE cladding). (Reproduced by permission of the *British Journal of Hospital Medicine*.)

The start of any laser treatment session should involve a certain set routine to avoid major problems with the equipment. For all but the most advanced YAG lasers it is immensely important to ensure that the water supply has been attached and is turned on, so that there is a free flow of clean water as and when the machine requires it. We make it an absolute rule that this is the first procedure to be performed by those responsible for the laser. The second

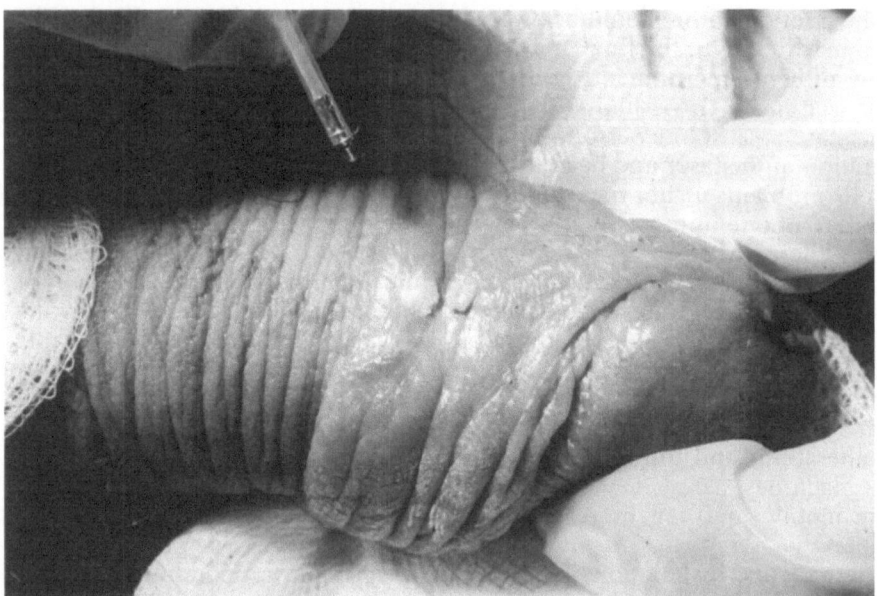

Fig. 2.3. A fibre delivery system with cooling of fibre tip by gas passing through outer "cannula".

manoeuvre is to turn on the electrical supply. The exact details of this will depend on the local arrangements, but most machines require a three-phase electrical circuit with 40 W power per phase, which is the type of circuit generally used to supply portable X-ray machines. Therefore it is likely that such a circuit will at least be close to a theatre if not already installed in the operating room. Next the machine can be turned on, usually by a key system. It is a good idea for the most frequent operators of the machine to have their own keys. In our practice one set of keys remains in the charge of the senior theatre nurse as a fail-safe mechanism. One further key is always kept available should all else fail.

Once the machine has been switched on, it is a good idea to let it run for a period to reach normal operating temperature. Most machines will benefit from running for approximately half an hour prior to use. However, in practice, we have been impressed by the stability of most machines even when circumstances require them to be switched on just before treatment.

The Fibre

The urologist should be familiar with the fibre he is going to use. In urological practice this is usually just a simple quartz glass fibre (Fig. 2.2). The central glass core is usually covered by a thin layer of a soft plastic and then a strong outer cladding of polytetrafluoroethylene (PTFE). Most other laser users will use a fibre of this basic construction but with the addition of a loose outer sheath of plastic, down which cooling gas is passed when the laser fibre is used in the atmosphere (Fig. 2.3). However, in urological practice cooling of the fibre from the surrounding irrigation fluid is usually sufficient and therefore this outer "cannula" is not necessary. Obviously if the laser is being used for open surgery of any sort, then a fibre with a cooling cannula will be required.

Recently the fibre manufacturers have actively promoted the use of disposable fibres which are prepared to a very high standard in the factory for single use. We still use a "repairable fibre" and each user must decide which is most appropriate for his practice. Urologists should certainly not be daunted by the problems of repairing fibres, assuming that they are using a sensible simple system consisting basically of the PTFE-clad fibre alone. In the early days of laser urology there were many systems with outer coverings of heavy material or even metal designed to protect the operating room staff by absorbing any escaping laser energy in the event of an unknown break in the fibre. However, this was a rather misguided development and most fibres are now of a much simpler design. The user should be warned, however, that many of this previous generation of fibres are not repairable in the operating room due to their complex construction, and require expensive repair at the manufacturer's plant.

A simple PTFE fibre can be prepared for use by removing a length of the outer PTFE coat with a suitable stripper provided by the manufacturer. An adequate length is one that will easily pass through the endoscope to be used. The inner layer of plastic should then be removed for a length of 1-1½ cm from the end of the fibre and finally any remaining vestiges of silicone can be removed with a soft optical polishing cloth or alternatively yet another specific device supplied with the fibre. It is important not to damage the fibre during this process, since this will lead to some loss of laser energy.

The Cleave

Preparing the fibre is the subject of much anxiety and mystique. However, there is no more to it than cutting glass or tiles. The essential tool is a good-quality cutting blade such as a tungsten carbide blade, which can be lightly drawn across one surface of the fibre, thereby scoring it. It is then necessary to break the fibre sharply at this point using the fingers. If the proximal end of the fibre launch delivery mechanism is inserted into the laser aperture on the machine, a red helium–neon aiming beam should be visible. If the spot of light from the newly cleaved fibre end is perfectly round when the fibre is held perpendicular to a suitable surface, then the cleave is satisfactory. In practice a small amount of irregularity in this spot is acceptable, but we would recommend that a good cleave is achieved at the start of each patient session. This does tend to come with practice. When we started these procedures, we used several feet of fibre per month, but now a 3-metre fibre length lasts for over a year – barring accidents such as the theatre trolleys running over the fibre or one's colleagues stamping their feet on it!

There is no doubt, however, that in much of the world the disposable fibre system will be the system of choice. The fibres should come prepacked and sterilised from the manufacturer and can be simply plugged into the laser aperture on the machine and disposed of afterwards.

Calibration

Each manufacturer will give specific recommendations for calibration of its laser prior to a treatment session, and these should be adhered to rigidly. Most YAG lasers will have a wide range of possible power emissions, but will generally be most stable over a particular part of the total possible range depending on how the manufacturer has adjusted the machine. It is therefore worth asking the service engineer to set the laser to work most efficiently at the power range you expect to use most frequently.

The choice of powers for laser coagulation will be learnt by experience, and you should be prepared to adjust both power and duration of radiation according to the clinical situation and in particular according to the response seen in the irradiated tissues. There are certain guidelines that may help the beginner, though, and these are included in the detailed discussions of particular techniques. As a very general guideline, a power of 15–20 W is a suitable starting point for urethral and ureteric lasering and 40 W for lasering within the bladder.

The next step is to ensure that the equipment is available to allow the safe use of the laser via an endoscope. In most cases the procedure during which the laser is to be used will be endoscopic and the surgeon's eye must be protected from the effects of any reflected laser light by an add-on eyepiece of KG3 glass which will selectively absorb the YAG laser wavelength. An alternative method is to use a video camera and to operate using the image on a conveniently situated TV screen. Those not completely familiar with this technique can use a beam splitter system that allows both the TV image and the surgeon's eye view to be available. However, it is necessary to check with the video manufacturer that a suitable filter has been fitted to the camera system to allow the surgeon to look down the beam splitter at the site of laser action without danger. If a laser is being used with an endoscope sufficiently often, then it may be worth getting the manufacturer to insert a protective lens as part of the structure of the endoscope. This has the great advantage of avoiding the misting that often occurs between the add-on eyepiece and the original eyepiece of the instrument.

The final option is the use of protective goggles, but most endoscopic surgery is almost impossible to perform whilst wearing them. They also have the disadvantage of being relatively expensive. However, they are essential should the laser be fired in the operating room for open surgery such as the treatment of warts. In such cases only the minimum staff required should be in the room and all those present, including the patient, should wear goggles. Since goggles protective against YAG and argon laser light can appear similar it is important where both types of laser are being used in the same environment that the goggles are labelled with their protective characteristics and checked before use to avoid mistakes.

Instruments

The appropriate endoscopes should be available. Although fibres can be passed down the standard operating channels of most urological instruments, there is a risk of damaging the carefully prepared cleaved end of the fibre. Therefore the major instrument manufacturers have produced modified laser inserts

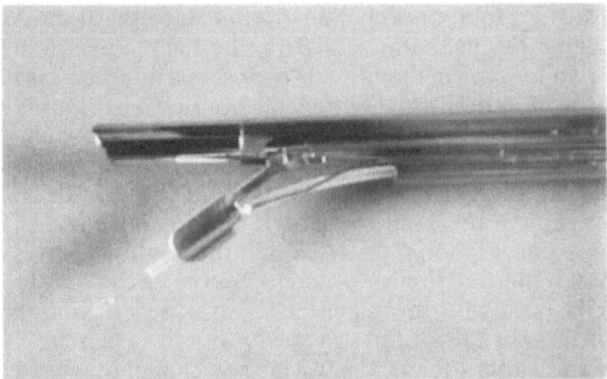

Fig. 2.4. A fibre passing through a modified Albarran lever which traps the fibre, keeping it under control as it leaves the cystoscope (Storz, Rimmer Bros., London).

which have a protective channel for the fibre. By all means use instruments with an ordinary working channel if necessary, but do check that the fibre can be easily passed through them without damage.

In our practice we use a cystoscope with a modified Albarran lever which traps the distal end of the fibre keeping it nicely under control (Fig. 2.4). The urethrotome is used for most urethral laser surgery. We have found it best to use it with the knife left in position to reduce leakage from the instrument; care is of course necessary about the knife. McPhee introduced a modified resectoscope (Storz; Fig. 2.5) which includes in the working element both a traditional loop and a separate channel which carries a laser fibre. The channel directs the laser fibre so that it passes just within the loop. This has the advantage of allowing resection followed immediately by laser coagulation without having to change instruments.

Final Preparations

At this stage the machine should be running but disabled, so that accidental firing of the laser is impossible. We have a strict rule that the machine remains disabled until the endoscope is within the patient, the fibre has been passed

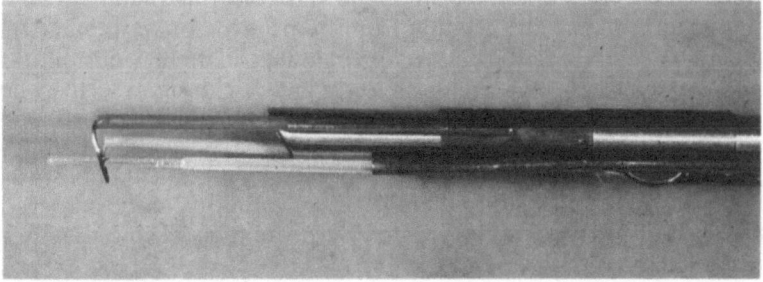

Fig. 2.5. Combined resectoscope and channel for urological laser fibre (McPhee design, Storz instrument, Rimmer Bros., London).

through it, and all is ready for coagulation to begin. At that stage the laser is enabled and the surgeon thereafter has control of firing by means of a foot pedal. Should the surgeon wish to remove the fibre or endoscope, then he asks for the laser to be disabled. In addition the theatre staff are now sufficiently familiar with the laser to disable it themselves should the surgeon remove the endoscope without formally requesting the disabling to be performed. Disabling in most machines should be a simple matter of pressing one button which leaves the laser on standby ready to be enabled again at a moment's notice.

The final preparation before coagulation is to check that the aiming beam is on the target. The YAG laser light is invisible and therefore a low-power helium–neon (HeNe) laser is built into the machine to provide an aiming beam visible to the operator. The beams of the two lasers should be carefully aligned so that there is no significant difference between the beam paths. If for any reason the red spot of the aiming beam laser is not visible, there is no means of knowing where the YAG laser energy is going to be directed and lasering is not safe. Although it may be suspected that the aiming beam has inadvertently been directed elsewhere, the other possibility is that there is a malfunction in the system, or indeed a break in the fibre so that the laser energy may be escaping. We therefore have an absolute rule of "no HeNe – no lasering". So just prior to coagulation the spot is put on the target and subsequent coagulation is performed according to the requirements of the clinical situation.

Techniques

Coagulation of Superficial Bladder Cancer

After a full examination of the bladder, biopsies are done if necessary. This pathological assessment of the depth of invasion can, arguably, be sacrificed in laser coagulation of small, apparently superficial tumours but should certainly not be omitted in the assessment of a patient presenting with his first tumour. The whole process should be done with the bladder minimally distended, just sufficient to open out all the "nooks and crannies". Overdistension will reduce the thickness of the bladder wall, increasing the possibility of onward transmission of the laser energy, and will be uncomfortable for the patient.

It is very important to stop all bleeding from biopsies before commencing lasering. Whilst the YAG laser can be used for coagulation, in our opinion it is much easier to stop the bleeding with a diathermy electrode or the resectoscope loop prior to insertion of the laser fibre. The use of coagulating insulated biopsy forceps is ideal, particularly if multiple biopsies have been taken. Once haemorrhage is under control lasering can proceed. Ideally all haemostasis should be completed so that the subsequent laser coagulation can be achieved in one session without having to remove the laser fibre and disable the laser repeatedly.

The fibre is passed down the instrument channel and the operator should get close to the target tissue and pass the fibre through the endoscope so that the distal tip of the laser fibre can be seen as well as the red aiming beam spot.

If you are too far away, then this spot will be difficult to see, particularly if the albarran lever is pointing the fibre tip away from the target. It may also be difficult to see if high-power light sources are being used to allow video recording. It may help if the light intensity is reduced temporarily to allow the aiming beam spot to be seen.

The fibre is best held 2–3 mm away from the tissue and a pulse of laser energy is fired at the target. Should the effect be minimal then it is necessary to get closer or increase the power. On the other hand if the effect is too vigorous, with disruption of the surface, then the cystoscope and laser fibre should be withdrawn further from the target (or the power reduced) and the pulse repeated to assess the effect again. There is a certain knack in being able to keep the fibre quite close to the tissue despite the patient's respiratory movements and one's own movements. It is quite frequently the case that small amounts of tissue debris attach to the end of the fibre as it gets warmer; these can usually be cleaned off by drawing the fibre back through the albarran lever a few centimetres. Should this manoeuvre fail, the laser may have to be disabled, and the fibre withdrawn entirely and cleaned with a swab.

We approach superficial bladder tumours by using the laser set at 40–45 W and firing 2–4 second bursts of laser energy at the base of the tumour, particularly if it is a polypoid tumour. Should the tumour be sessile coagulation is first done peripherally, around the tumour, and then centrally on the tumour mass. Should no effect be seen it is necessary to get closer to the tumour or increase the power or the pulse duration. Conversely should the effects be too vigorous the instrument and fibre need to be pulled back and the pulse duration or power reduced – or sometimes a combination of all three. It is quite surprising how the absorption of different areas of the bladder might vary and inflamed vascular areas will appear to absorb vigorously. Blood if present will avidly absorb energy – so much so that little microexplosions develop. This has the disadvantage of often causing more bleeding and leading to extra debris floating in the bladder which tends to stick to the fibre end.

Adequate laser coagulation leads to a visible shrinkage of tissue followed by the tumour seeming to rise up from the surrounding mucosa and blanching in a characteristic way that signifies protein denaturation and adequate coagulation (Fig. 2.6). This, in general terms, may appear similar to the coagulative effects of cystodiathermy but without the "boiling" effect of bubble formation and release of debris. If the laser is too close or the power is too great, it may burn a hole, especially if the fibre touches the tissue. This may also damage the fibre end. A bright flash tends to be seen if the tissue is touched with the end of the fibre and afterwards a small pin-hole perforation; this is usually of no consequence.

Larger tumours can be more difficult to coagulate completely, particularly the part of the tumour farthest away from the operator. Experience will show that repositioning the endoscope, with increased or decreased distension of the bladder and sometimes manual pressure suprapubically, will allow adequate access to the tumour site. Tumours in certain positions such as at the bladder neck can be difficult to reach and here the resectoscope may be required anyway, after which coagulation of the site may be possible.

In very large exophytic tumours the coagulated exophytic mass can be removed by brushing it off with the endoscope, the fibre or biopsy forceps. In fact biopsy at this stage may still give the pathologist a tissue specimen from

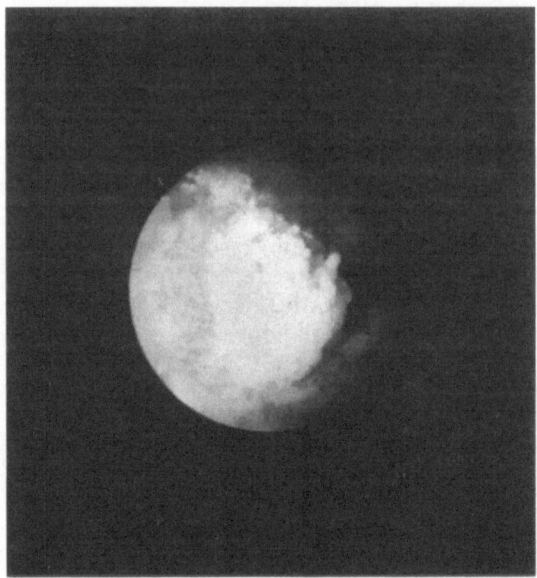

Fig. 2.6. Bladder cancer partially coagulated by YAG laser. (Reproduced by permission of the *British Journal of Hospital Medicine.*)

which the nature of the tumour and its grade can be assessed. However, large exophytic tumour masses should be resected first and coagulated with the laser subsequently. As described above, laser coagulation should be preceded by good haemostasis. This may mean that after an extensive resection coagulation needs to be delayed for a few days.

We do not routinely drain bladders after laser treatment alone. However, if large tumours have been resected and large areas coagulated with the laser then bladder drainage by catheter may be required. We do drain bladders where tumour in a diverticulum has been coagulated.

Invasive Bladder Cancer

Treatment of invasive tumours involves a conventional resection of the initial tumour deep enough for adequate staging. Subsequent laser irradiation is carried out after an interval of about 1 week when adherent blood clot has lysed.

A higher power than is generally used for superficial tumours (45–50 W) is applied in 4–5-second pulses to ensure treatment to the entire tumour and surrounding mucosa. The characteristic blanching is less apparent in a previously resected field, so particular care has to be taken to ensure even irradiation of the whole target area.

Flexible Cystoscopy and Laser Therapy

The clinician needs to justify the treatment of superficial tumours by an expensive laser coagulator rather than cheap, conventional and undoubtedly effective diathermy. We have found that laser treatment in combination with flexible cystoscopy allows almost all of our patients with low-grade superficial bladder cancer (who comprise about 80% of all bladder cancer patients) to be managed entirely as outpatients using only topical urethral anaesthesia. The savings in terms of bed occupancy, theatre and anaesthetic costs can be considerable, particularly if the laser is sited in a multi-disciplinary endoscopy unit where its use, and costs, can be shared with other users (primarily gastroenterologists and chest physicians). The minimal need for catheterisation post-operatively can further reduce costs.

There are also clear medical advantages for the many patients who are relatively elderly and unfit and who would otherwise require repeated anaesthetics over many years. As long as the procedure is adequately explained, few patients given the choice will opt for conventional inpatient treatment (Flannigan et al. 1988). Those that do are usually elderly women who can find the flexible procedure somewhat embarrassing, or those whose fear of discomfort during treatment is extreme.

It is of course possible to use fine diathermy electrodes with flexible cystoscopes, but these are distinctly uncomfortable, particularly on the trigone. The technique usually necessitates parenteral analgesia and sedation, which seems to negate the major advantage of flexible cystoscopy. Also, many flexible instruments are not built to allow the safe use of diathermy and there is the remote risk of current leak to the operator's eye.

Patients on the waiting list for annual check cystoscopy for the surveillance of transitional cell cancer of the bladder make up a large proportion of the operating lists of any urological department, committing much of the available surgical, anaesthetic and nursing resources. However, it has been shown that 60%–80% of diagnostic or surveillance "check cystoscopies" do not require the performance of any operative procedure beyond the insertion of the cystoscope itself. Recent developments, especially the availability of flexible fibre-optic cystoscopes, and the current need to improve the efficiency of treatment in the presence of diminishing or re-allocated resources, have led to the possibility of changes in the management of this patient population. Using topical urethral anaesthesia alone the latest flexible cystoscopes allow the accurate, easy and painless "outpatient" assessment of the lower urinary tract.

In 1985 we set out to determine whether we could continue surveillance of, and add treatment for, all lower-risk bladder cancer patients (the "yearly check cystoscopy") in an outpatient setting, with appropriate planned admission and general anaesthetic only for those shown to require it. Of 84 patients assessed as suitable 79 (94%) successfully underwent cystoscopy in an outpatient setting using local urethral anaesthesia alone. Biopsy and YAG laser coagulation of superficial bladder cancer were found to be possible and acceptable in 12 of the 13 patients with tumours (one refused treatment).

Since this was then a new treatment method these patients were initially re-examined as outpatients between 4 and 6 weeks later to ensure adequate tumour destruction. Once confidence was established in the technique we reverted to standard follow-up routines, with the difference that they occurred in an outpatient setting. At the repeat cystoscopy coagulation was found to be complete in 8 patients, leaving a healing ulcerated area. One patient was thought to be incompletely treated and required additional laser coagulation. Those with low-grade and solitary tumours that had been adequately treated were booked for a repeat flexible endoscopy 1 year later. No patient refused either the offer of repeat flexible endoscopy or further laser treatment.

Overall 75 patients (92.5%) were entirely managed as outpatients. The method therefore reduces the need for general anaesthesia in this largely elderly population and allows the more efficient use of departmental resources.

Method: Flexible Cystoscopy

It is wise initially to select for screening by outpatient flexible cystoscopy those patients with a low risk of tumour recurrence, superficial ($pT_a–pT_1$), low-grade ($G_1–G_2$) disease or who are at high risk of complications from general anaesthesia. Once the confidence has been gained to extend the procedure to include tumour treatment, then a wider patient population can be screened.

In our practice all procedures were performed at a clinic held during one 3-hour morning session a week, staffed by one urologist and one nurse with shared secretarial help to deal with bookings and reports. Six patients per session were initially booked in, though greater experience allowed up to 10 to be seen later.

On arrival informed consent for cystoscopy, followed by biopsy and treatment if necessary, was obtained from each patient. In males urethral anaesthesia was achieved by the instillation of 20 ml lignocaine jelly down the urethra with 10 minutes' delay (by the clock) whilst it became effective. During this time the cystoscope was being prepared by immersion in activated glutaraldehyde solution for 10 minutes. One flexible endoscope is sufficient, though a second will increase throughput.

The operator questioned and examined the patient and explained the procedure further. For females lubricant jelly was applied just to the tip of the endoscope and to the urethra. After rinsing off the sterilising solution (including washing out the irrigating channel) the cystoscope was passed down the urethra under direct vision. Once in the bladder a systematic examination was performed to ensure inspection of all areas. The ability to flex the distal tip of the endoscope back on itself allows a good vision of the whole of the bladder neck, internal meatus and the anterior wall of the bladder.

Once the endoscopist becomes accustomed to the rather different view obtained using the flexible instrument and the manipulations necessary to obtain a satisfactory view of all parts of the bladder then the accuracy of cystoscopy appears high (Fowler et al. 1984; Powell et al. 1984; Clayman et al. 1984). Our own pilot study confirmed accuracy and allowed us to become familiar with the instrument; we would recommend this procedure in the initial stages, particularly if the endoscopist is unfamiliar with flexible endoscopes generally (gastroscopes etc.). The image differs both in quality, being slightly granular as a result of the fibre bundles making up the image, and in orientation. The rigid cystoscope is usually lying in the centre of the bladder and has an angle of view offset by 30° to 70° from the "straight ahead" long axis of the instrument. The flexiscope tends to lie or "creep" along the lower surface of the bladder and the view is directly ahead from the tip of the scope.

Method: Laser Coagulation

The patients in whom small recurrences were found were biopsied followed by tumour coagulation using a YAG laser (Pilkington Medical Systems (now Living Technology plc) Fiberlase 100).

The YAG laser energy is transmitted along a 0.4-mm (400-μm) diameter quartz glass fibre passed down the instrument channel of the endoscope. Larger standard 0.6-mm fibres are much more rigid and significantly reduce the mobility of the tip of the endoscope, with the result that some tumours at the bladder neck especially will be inaccessible. The quartz glass fibre should be disinfected by soap and water cleaning followed by immersion of the distal 3–4 m of fibre coiled up in a standard tray containing activated glutaraldehyde.

It is essential to place the relatively unprotected "urological" fibre within a protective sheath or cannula so that the sharp fibre tip does not protrude during its passage down the instrument channel and damage the channel's inner lining. Such damage is most likely to occur where the side arm entry port of the instrument channel meets the main body of the endoscope and at the distal bending section of the instrument. If this does happen the results can be expensive, particularly if the internal damage goes unnoticed and is followed by further immersion in disinfecting solutions! It is often best and easiest to pass the fibre with the endoscope tip pointing straight ahead in the bladder. This position is much easier to determine in some manufacturers' instruments than in others.

A certain dexterity and a helping hand from an assistant is useful at this point to achieve rapid replacement of the biopsy forceps (if used) by the fibre to allow rapid coagulation, especially if bleeding from the biopsy site is marked. Treatment itself is essentially just as for laser coagulation using a rigid cystoscope, but with two provisos. First, distension of the bladder must be avoided as there is no quicker way of losing the patient's cooperation. Second, the laser should be fired in short bursts of 0.5–1.0 seconds, repeated until the target tumour is completely coagulated as determined by the characteristic shrinkage and blanching of the target tissue.

Most patients are aware of the laser energy and usually describe it as a suprapubic burning or stinging sensation which is rarely uncomfortable as long as short pulses are given with an interval of several seconds between each to permit heat dispersal. We use a laser power of 30–40 W with a pulse duration of 0.5–1 seconds. It is most convenient to set the instrument panel timer to a longer exposure and to control the pulse length with the foot pedal.

The fibre is stroked linearly across the tumour at a distance of 2–3 mm from it. About 2–3 seconds' total exposure on each area is enough to produce the blanching effect which indicates that an adequate depth of coagulation has been achieved. Some authorities (e.g. Hofstetter 1987) recommend first treating a ring of normal mucosa approximately 0.5 cm in radius around the tumour to seal off lymphatics and small blood vessels. The theoretical benefits of this, as discussed later, are probably greater than the practical ones and as the laser effect spreads for some distance beyond the irradiated area this is probably overtreatment.

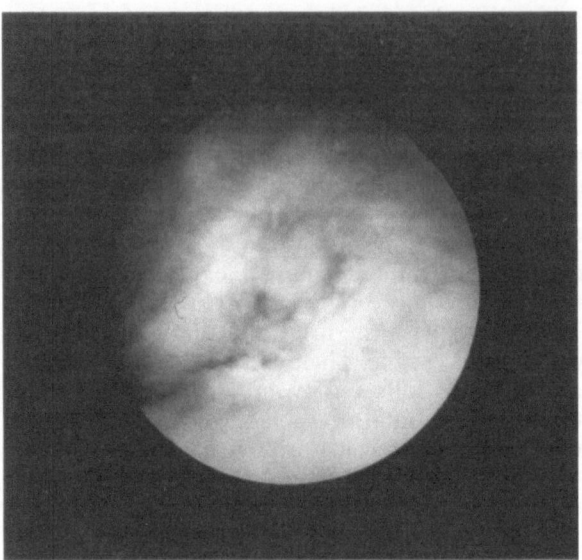

Fig. 2.7. Site of laser-treated bladder tumour 6 weeks after treatment showing healing ulcer.

Precise control of the fibre tip is less easy with flexible than with rigid endoscopes, particularly when a significant angulation is necessary to reach the tumour. In addition the flexible endoscope naturally lies along the bladder wall so that there is a tendency to approach tumours obliquely. Therefore the laser energy reaching the furthermost part of a sizeable tumour may be inadequate. In these situations it is quite safe to exceed the normal power as the tangential incidence of the beam reduces the energy density considerably. It is our policy to check such patients about a month later, when the adequately coagulated tumour will have sloughed, in case there is a small area of residual tumour which needs further treatment (Fig. 2.7).

As mentioned there may be several difficulties which relate to the fibre. The standard urology fibre is a bare 600-μm quartz fibre. This is stiff enough to restrict significantly the maximum angulation of the flexible cystoscope and can make for difficult access to tumours near the bladder neck which may have been easily seen previously. Often a "J" manoeuvre, approaching the bladder neck from above, will be successful but care must be taken to ensure that forward scatter of energy will not damage the emerging cystoscope. The increased flexibility of the newer 400-μm fibres largely alleviates this problem.

A more serious problem is that of damage to the endoscope by the fibre itself. The tip of the 600-μm fibre is sharp and stiff and in attempting to force it down a working channel thrown into a sharp bend by a serpentine prostatic urethra it is easy to impinge on and pierce the channel lining. Other potential sites of damage are, as mentioned above, where the angled side entry port joins the endoscope body and at the distal flexible tip (if this has not been straightened out in the bladder). A 400-μm fibre is only slightly better in this respect than is the 600-μm, but there are several solutions. One option is to withdraw the instrument into the straight penile urethra, insert the fibre, but not let it protrude, and advance again into the bladder. If use of the laser is expected the fibre can be prepositioned before introducing the cystoscope, though this significantly reduces irrigation flow, particularly with the 600-μm fibre. A second possibility is to insert the fibre coaxially inside and just short of the end of a piece of fine-bore tubing. The leading soft end of this introducer will guide the fibre safely round bends and can be withdrawn once the fibre is safely through the instrument and into the bladder. A variation on this theme is to use a gas-cooled fibre, with the gas turned off, as this has a coaxial sheath held by a blunt metal tip which is much less likely to damage the working channel lining than is a sharp bare fibre. Again though, its large size will all but abolish irrigant flow.

Flexible cystoscopes are several times more expensive than their rigid counterparts and particular care must be taken when using a laser to avoid damaging them. It should be self-evident that the laser must not be fired unless both the tip of the fibre and the helium–neon aiming spot are visible. It is not unknown for a 600-μm fibre to crack under extreme angulation and yet retain integrity due to the Teflon sheath until the laser is fired into the optical bundle. In this case the fibre tip will appear to manipulate normally but the aiming spot will be lost.

The back scatter of laser energy via the endoscope optics is a potential source of damage to the operator's retina, and a suitable filter should be fitted over the eyepiece. It is unnecessary for other participants to wear goggles as the laser will not be enabled until the fibre tip is inside the bladder.

After laser use all endoscopes should be leak tested, as if damage has been done this may be made irreparable by immersion in sterilising solutions.

Complications of Laser Treatment

The only significant complication of laser irradiation is the possibility of damaging an adjacent loop of bowel from forward scattering of energy through the bladder wall. This is most unlikely if the power is kept below 50 W. Hofstetter (1987) had only 3 patients out of more than 1000 in whom secondary intestinal perforation occurred, when too high a power (in excess of 80 W) was inadvertently delivered. Cos and Di Sant'Agnese (1988) found in dog bladder that bowel injury occurred with a 7-second irradiation (7 × 1-second pulses) at 60 W, or more than 10 seconds at 40 W. Irradiation for 7 seconds at 40 or 50 W produced a coagulative necrosis from 4 mm to full thickness. Although Cos and Di Sant'Agnese saw bladder perforation in some experimental animals treated at high doses it seems agreed by other authors that in the clinical setting the structural integrity of the bladder wall is maintained despite full-thickness damage, unlike the effect with diathermy. This consideration is probably irrelevant when dealing with superficial tumours. Also in contrast to electrical coagulation, obturator nerve stimulation is not seen with the laser.

It is prudent though, as well as considerate, to avoid thinning the bladder wall by any more distension than is required merely to unfold the mucosa. Vision is rarely a problem as there is no bleeding during treatment unless biopsies have been taken. Treating tumours in the dome, particularly in elderly women, is therefore quite safe. None of our patients has had noticeable secondary bleeding when the necrotic tumour separates a week or so later. One patient complained of frequency and dysuria, with sterile urine, for some days after extensive laser treatment, but we have seen no other significant problems.

Discussion

Whilst the initial aim of our study was to determine whether "outpatient" endoscopic assessment improved the efficient use of our resources by selecting patients requiring treatment which merited inpatient admission, it became obvious that a combination of painless outpatient endoscopy with effective treatment of localised, superficial tumour at the same session would be an attractive and reasonable proposition for some patients. The YAG laser proved to be an effective coagulator of bladder tumours.

Both our clinical experience and measurement of discomfort by using a visual analogue scale (VAS) scores (Huskisson 1974) suggest that laser coagulation is no more painful than taking a small endoscopic biopsy, and in some it is completely painless. This is particularly so if the laser is fired in short bursts of 0.5–1.0 seconds that are repeated until the target tumour is completely coagulated.

Comparison with diathermy coagulation is under way and there is no doubt in our minds that this is also quite well tolerated in many well-motivated patients. It is our strong impression that the laser coagulation is less painful and more acceptable overall. The ability to give multiple short-duration laser pulses seems to allow more reliable and complete coagulation. However, the capital costs of the YAG laser are high compared with diathermy equipment and we are assessing which is the more cost effective.

Other attempts to reduce the costs and inconvenience of cystoscopic surveillance for bladder cancer using general anaesthesia, such as the use of ultrasound (Malone et al. 1986) with or without urinary cytology, do not yet match the accuracy of directly viewing the interior of the bladder. The only possible exception is the cytological diagnosis of carcinoma in situ (Juul et al. 1986). In our view our arrangements are easier to establish and continue than those of the alternatives.

The patients benefit from a simple, painless, quick endoscopy without the disruption of hospital admission and the risks of general anaesthesia are avoided in what is generally an elderly group often suffering intercurrent diseases. The clinician and his unit benefit from the opportunity to plan the use of inpatient operating lists for patients known to require resection and inpatient resources. In addition, once the outpatient cystoscopy arrangements are established a proportion of the diagnostic cystoscopies can also be performed in this manner, particularly those presenting with microscopic haematuria and recurrent urinary infections, which allows further savings in inpatient resources.

One of the criticisms of laser coagulation is that inadequate material is available for histological examination, particularly in respect of determining tumour stage. Small cold-cup biopsies of the lesion can be taken through a flexible cystoscope prior to laser treatment which may be adequate for confirming the presence and grade of tumour, but the base cannot be adequately sampled. We feel strongly that a patient's initial tumour should be resected conventionally together with random biopsies and bimanual examination so that complete histological information is available at the start. Those patients with papillary low-grade superficial disease are then followed up on the outpatient laser list initially at 3 months and then at increasing intervals as long as they remain clear. Papillary recurrences are coagulated as they occur. Patients who develop sessile tumours, large numbers of recurrences or high-grade malignant cells on voided cytology revert to conventional treatment. So far this has not happened in our practice.

In this way the risk of significant understaging seems to be very low and large numbers of patients fall into the category in which routine histology is unnecessary. We rarely find large recurrences in this group, but if there is a significant exophytic growth the base is likely to be inadequately treated. After initial coagulation the denatured tumour may be detached with biopsy forceps and a second treatment given to the base. If this is not done the patient should be brought back in 3–4 weeks to check for residual tumour. This can be quite time consuming and we find that resection is more satisfactory for tumours larger than 2–3 cm.

Conclusions

The YAG laser in conjunction with flexible cystoscopy can make a useful contribution to the management of a large proportion of bladder cancer patients by enabling anaesthesia-free, outpatient treatment of their recurrences. As long as certain selection criteria are maintained there is no real risk of tumour understaging, and there may be a reduction in tumour recurrence rate after laser compared with electrical coagulation. The techniques are easy to learn and there are considerable benefits to be had in terms of convenience and economy, especially in a multispecialty laser unit.

References

Cos LR, Di Sant'Agnese PA (1988) Nd-YAG nomogram dosimetry scale for the bladder. J Urol 139:196–198

Clayman RV, Reddy P, Lange PH (1984) Flexible fibreoptic and rigid rod lens endoscopy of the lower urinary tract: a prospective controlled comparison. J Urol 131:715–716

Flannigan GM, Gelister JSK, Noble JG, Milroy EJG (1988) Rigid versus flexible cystoscopy. A controlled trial of patient tolerance. Br J Urol 62:537–540

Fowler CG, Badenoch DF, Thakar DR (1984) Practical experience with flexible fibrescope cystoscopy in outpatients. Br J Urol 56:618–621

Hofstetter AG (1987) Neodymium:YAG laser treatment of bladder tumours. J Endourol 1:115–117

Huskisson EC (1974) The measurement of pain. Lancet ii:1127–1131

Juul N, Torp-Pedersen S, Larsen S, Rasmussen F, Holm HH (1986) Bladder tumour control by abdominal ultrasound and urine cytology. Scand J Urol Nephrol 20:275–278

Malone PR, Weston-Underwood J, Aron PM, Wilkinson KW, Joseph AEA, Riddle PR (1986) The use of transabdominal ultrasound in the detection of early B1 tumours. Br J Urol 51:520–522

Powell PH, Manohar V, Ramsden PD, Hall RR (1984) A flexible cystoscope. Br J Urol 56:622–624

Chapter 3

Laser Treatment of Urological Tumours 1: Transitional Cell Tumours

T. A. McNicholas and A. J. Pope

Bladder Tumours

There has been enormous interest in the possibility that endoscopic neodymium yttrium aluminium garnet (YAG) laser coagulation could add to the management of bladder cancer.

Most patients present with superficial disease not involving the muscle of the bladder wall (T_a, T_1: UICC 1978) and whilst their life expectancy may be good compared with those presenting with muscle invasive disease, some 55% will suffer recurrences by 3 years and 25% of those with stage T_1 tumours will have progressed to develop muscle invasive disease by 2 years after diagnosis (Cutler et al. 1982). Once diagnosed these patients will thereafter require long-term surveillance with cystoscopy and the repeated treatment of small, superficial transitional cell tumours of the bladder. An endoscopic method that could reduce the incidence of recurrence and subsequent invasion would be welcome, particularly if it could also contribute to the control of invasive disease once present.

Standard treatment consists of biopsy and either coagulation with the coagulating diathermy electrode passed through the cystoscope or transurethral (electro)resection of the bladder tumour (TURB) with the resectoscope. TURB alone is predictably curative only for those presenting with superficial disease. Full thickness bladder wall removal by TURB results in gross urinary extravasation; thus reliable endoscopic management of bladder tumours deeply invading the muscle of the bladder wall is not possible using conventional techniques.

Historical Background

The first workers to apply laser energy to the bladder were Parsons et al. (1966), who exposed an opened canine bladder to 694-nm light from a pulsed ruby laser, using energy levels of 10–15 J. The histological appearances after 3–10 days showed minor damage confined to the mucosa with sharp transition from neighbouring normal tissue. Parsons et al. suggested that this new energy modality might destroy the bladder cancer endoscopically, provided a suitable "light pipe" could be found. This breakthrough did not come until the development of the flexible quartz fibre (Nath et al. 1973).

Earlier, Mulvaney and Beck (1968) had studied the in vitro effects of both ruby and CO_2 lasers on urinary calculi and had achieved partial disintegration with a pulsed beam. They commented that neither laser was the ideal for the destruction of tumours, and suggested that the newly developed argon laser might be more suitable.

First reports of the argon laser's urological applications soon followed (Staehler et al. 1976). Although it has found great use in other branches of medicine the argon laser is not ideal for urology as it is low-powered, poorly haemostatic and, although readily transmitted by quartz glass fibres, only penetrates tissue for 1–2 mm. As the blue-green argon laser light is well absorbed by haemoglobin it may theoretically be ideal for treating pigmented lesions such as haemangiomas; but although effective for small bladder tumours (Smith and Dixon 1984), in clinical practice it has been supplanted by the YAG laser.

The argon laser pumping a rhodamine B dye laser emits red light at 630 nm and is the standard light source for photodynamic therapy (Benson 1988). This promising technique involves the administration of photosensitisers which are retained selectively by tumour cells and cause a cytotoxic photochemical effect when exposed to specific wavelengths of light. Even in this field, though, the argon–dye laser is likely to be superseded by the newer, more powerful pulsed metal vapour lasers.

Mussiggang and Katsaros (1971) were the first to describe the use of the YAG laser for urological purposes. They realised its advantage over the CO_2 laser in that its output is transmissible via flexible glass fibres, and designed a prototype laser cystoscope using bundles of thin glass fibres to transmit the energy. Unfortunately the glass caused significant transmission losses and the resultant heat quickly melted the adhesive used to hold the bundles together unless the whole apparatus was water cooled. Mussiggang and Katsaros studied the effect of the pulsed YAG laser on bladder, prostate and renal tissue as well as on calculi. In the bladder they were able to produce coagulation to a depth of about 1 mm using a power of 25 W. This damage was sharply demarcated from the surrounding normal tissue. Staehler and Hofstetter (1979), using a power of 40 W for 2 seconds, produced full-thickness lesions (2–3 mm) in a rabbit bladder; by comparison an argon laser made shallower lesions.

The YAG laser has proved the best suited to the urologist's needs. It is most effective as a thermal coagulator and has been used successfully to treat lesions from the external genitalia to the renal pelvis. Good transmission through water, deep tissue penetration and excellent haemostatic properties make it the laser of choice for bladder cancer. It is in this field that most expertise has been gained, notably from European centres such as Oslo (Beisland and Seland

1986), and Munich where Hofstetter's group have treated over 1000 patients since 1976 (Hofstetter 1987).

So despite early interest in the argon laser it has become clear that for most purposes the YAG laser will fulfil the urologist's requirements and there is no economic justification for both types of laser in any but the most laser-orientated research units particularly those using argon as part of a photodynamic therapy (PDT) programme (see Chap. 6).

Certain YAG laser specifications used under controlled circumstances allow a more or less transmural thermal coagulation of the bladder wall without injury to adjacent organs. In fresh (in vitro) human bladder experiments 50 W YAG laser energy applied for 4 seconds raised the temperature of the outer bladder wall to 65 °C – enough to produce a full-thickness thermal necrosis – but adjacent loops of small bowel were not heated beyond 45 °C (Hofstetter and Frank 1980). For a given power of 40–50 W for 3–4 seconds in bladder a penetration to a depth of 3–6 mm has been described by Pensel et al. (1981), though others have found a lower penetration (Stein 1986; Smith and Landau 1989).

Stein described a series of experiments in which he assessed the depth of penetration of the YAG laser in an animal model and found the maximal depth of effect to be 2.62 mm at a power of 50 W for 4 seconds. The bladder was removed and examined immediately after laser exposure and this almost certainly led to an underestimate of the depth of the pathological injury. In our laboratories we have found 4–5 days to be the optimum time after injury to assess the maximal extent of damage (Bown et al. 1980).

We studied the lesions produced by the YAG laser on pig bladder and compared them with those produced by similar energies of diathermy current delivered through either a standard resectoscope loop or a coagulating electrode. The laser fibre was inserted at cystotomy to achieve a perpendicular incidence on the bladder mucosa. Powers of 20–60 W for 2 or 4 seconds were employed. In addition an area of mucosa of about 0.5 cm² was irradiated until the characteristic blanching which is normally taken as the end point in clinical use was achieved. The amount of bladder distension and the spot size (2 mm) were constant. Diathermy current was delivered by a computer-controlled generator with a feedback circuit so that a given amount of energy could be delivered in a specified time. Histological examination was performed at 5 days and the depth of lesion calculated from sections stained with haematoxylin and eosin and viewed using a microscope with a graticule eyepiece.

We found that at equal energy parameters the coagulation effect from the YAG laser was deeper than that produced by diathermy, though both modalities would achieve a full-thickness lesion in the relatively thin "minipig" bladder (mean thickness 2.6 mm) using powers of 40 W or more for in excess of 2 seconds. After laser treatment, the endoscopic appearances of "white coagulation" reliably signified a coagulation depth greater than 2 mm, and usually 3 mm, whereas the coagulation resulting from diathermy with the resectoscope loop was superficial, extending only 1–2 mm into the bladder wall (Pope and McNicholas 1989).

The diathermy electrode produced a similar depth of penetration to the laser for a given energy but there appeared to be a qualitative difference between the effects of the laser, which caused protein denaturation with little alteration of

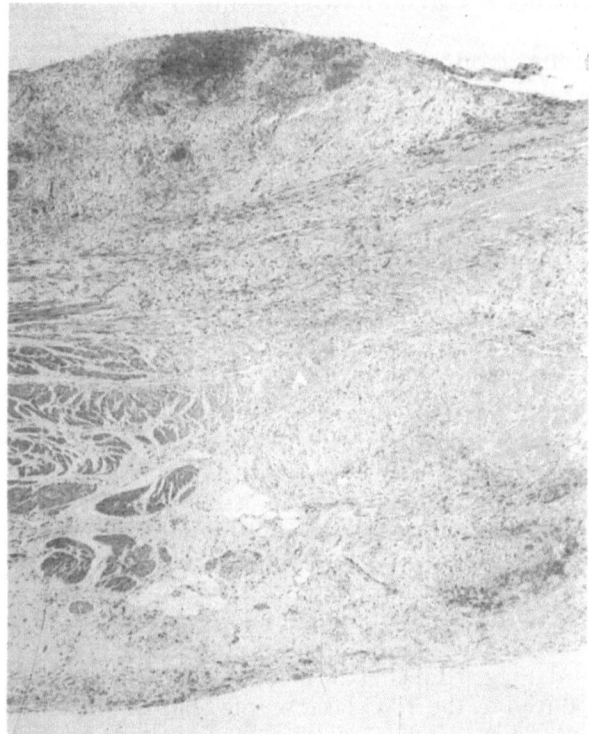

Fig. 3.1. Effect of YAG laser coagulation at 60 W for 4 seconds on pig bladder. (By courtesy of Mr. A. Pope)

the tissue architecture (Fig. 3.1), and of diathermy where more structural disruption could be seen (Fig. 3.2).

It is our distinct impression that conditions in the "real world", as opposed to the laboratory, are such that in practice the penetration depth will generally be less in the intact bladder and will also depend on the degree of bladder distension, which will alter the thickness of the bladder wall. In clinical practice it is safest, therefore, to avoid excessive distension of the bladder during treatment, even though there is a margin for safety.

Because the bladder wall appears to maintain its architectural integrity even after transmural laser treatment, definitive laser treatment of muscle-invading bladder tumours is theoretically feasible. YAG laser coagulation is claimed to improve results because of:

1. The greater depth and uniformity of coagulation of the bladder wall compared with that achieved by diathermy (Hofstetter and Frank 1980).

2. The early coagulation and therefore occlusion of lymphatic channels within the bladder (Zimmerman et al. 1984), which was shown in experimental studies using Indian ink injected into the dome of the rat bladder. The relevance of this to the human bladder can be questioned, and in our own attempts to reproduce these experiments we found that passage of the ink to the draining lymph nodes could be prevented by coagulating a rim of bladder surrounding the ink collection with either the YAG laser or diathermy electrocoagulation.

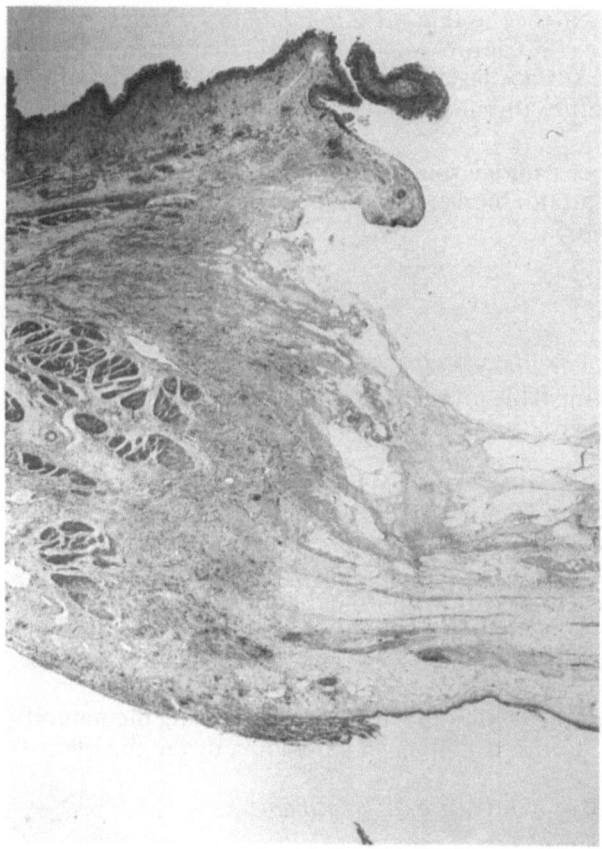

Fig. 3.2. Effect of diathermy electrode coagulation at 60 W for 4 seconds on pig bladder. (By courtesy of Mr. A. Pope)

The only marked difference was that diathermy coagulation more often led to subsequent necrotic rupture of the bladder dome with the late release of the ink to the nodes whereas the laser coagulated bladders remained intact.

3. Better haemostasis, which allows treatment without the necessity for post-operative catheterisation. This is certainly true for the smaller tumours and for many of the larger tumours if the target has been undisturbed during treatment. However, bleeding after biopsy can be troublesome, especially if using a flexible cystoscope with a limited irrigant flow rate.

If laser treatment follows extensive resection then in practice it is difficult to ensure haemostasis and focal bleeding points are best stopped by the resectoscope using the combination of coaptive pressure and diathermy to the bleeding vessel.

The YAG laser has theoretical advantages for more diffuse bleeding such as that following radiotherapy or from extensive ulcerating tumour but, again, in practice it is technically difficult to coagulate effectively what might be a large surface area. This will certainly take time and requires obsessional care from the operator. He should remember that the YAG laser energy will be widely scattered from the point of incidence so that the 2 mm or so spot size seen on the mucosa will cause a tissue effect approximately 4–6 mm in diameter; so he can reassure himself that the surface laser effect is therefore at least as widespread as that from the diathermy alternatives, whether loop or "rolly ball", and may be qualitatively better.

4. Less electrical interference with neuromuscular function. There is thus no danger from inadvertent obturator nerve stimulation when using the laser posterolaterally in the bladder.

Superficial Bladder Cancer

Clearly the influence of inadequate initial treatment and the presence of a widespread "field change" in unstable urothelium will have an influence on all results, particularly with regard to "recurrence" rates, whatever treatment modality is used.

When considering whether a particular treatment has the potential to reduce disease recurrence there are two features of "recurrence" to consider: firstly, tumour recurrence in the previously treated area (as accurately as this can be determined); secondly the "new occurrence" of tumour elsewhere in the bladder. Obviously differentiating these can be difficult if not impossible and generally "total" recurrence rates are reported rather than the incidence of recurrences at the site of the original treatment compared with recurrences or occurrences elsewhere.

At this point it may be helpful to review the literature concerning the natural history of (primarily superficial) transitional cell carcinoma of the bladder.

Natural History and Results of Conventional Treatment

Heney et al. (1982) described 353 cases of bladder cancer followed up by the surveillance of the National Bladder Cancer Collaborative Group A (NBCCG-A). One hundred and forty-eight of these patients were presenting with bladder cancer for the first time. Of these, 96 (65%) had superficial (T_a or T_1) disease, 48 (32%) had muscle invasive disease and 4 (2.7%) had metastases. After exclusions due to treatment with chemotherapy or short follow-up, 58 cases of superficial disease with a mean follow-up period of 74.8 months were described. Low risk of recurrence was found to be associated with small size (less than 3 cm diameter), grade 1 tumours, T_a stage, negative cytology, single tumours and normal random biopsies ("cystitis" being regarded as "normal" for the purposes of this study). Conversely, high risk of recurrence was associated with multiple tumours, diameter over 3 cm, grade 2–3 tumours, T_1 stage, positive cytology and abnormal random biopsies.

Cutler et al. (1982), reporting further NBCCG-A data, described 850 cases recruited between 1974 and 1976. Of these, 404 were presenting for the first time and 446 were known to have previously had bladder cancer. Their study showed an overall recurrence rate following conventional treatment for T_a tumours of 31% at 12 months, 45% at 24 months and 54% at 36 months, compared with 39%, 52% and 56% respectively for T_1 tumours. However, many other reports combine T_a and T_1 tumours. If this is done with Cutler et al.'s data an overall first-year recurrence rate of 34% is obtained, with 47% and 55%

at 24 and 36 months respectively.

Of course T_a and T_1 disease carry quite different prognoses. This same study indicated that T_a disease carried a 3% chance of progression to muscle invasion at 2 years compared with 25% for T_1 tumours.

Boyd and Burnand (1974) and Page et al. (1978) showed that the commonest sites of recurrences were at the dome and the anterior bladder wall whereas the original tumour was most commonly situated on the trigone, lateral and posterior walls of the bladder. Heney et al. (1982) stated that in 5.2% of new cases tumours were located in the dome, compared with 59% of patients having recurrent tumours at the dome.

Whilst it is generally agreed that some patients have multifocal disease, with a generally unstable urothelium, these reports do suggest, in addition to the "field effect", a different distribution of recurrent compared with initial tumours. This is possibly as a result of the implantation of cells released by the original treatment on to mucosa damaged by abrasion from the instrument used (Weldon and Soloway 1975), or of thermal injury from hot gases released during resection/coagulation rising to the dome (Heney et al. 1982).

On the other hand, in the study of Heney et al. (1982) random biopsy sites did not show any apparent increase in tumour development, and these must be regarded as damaged areas likely to be seeded. The authors suggested that these areas are normally coagulated following biopsy and that this produces an unhealthy environment for cells to seed on and to remain viable. The experimental evidence for this suggestion is weak. Soloway and Masters (1980) showed a marked increase in tumour cell implantation on areas of diathermy fulguration in the mouse bladder, supporting the concept of implantation as an important part of the aetiology of recurrent tumours. The mice were divided into two groups. One group underwent electrocautery of the dome of the bladder and the other group had no interference with their bladders; both groups then had a cell suspension of a FANFT-induced murine transitional cell tumour introduced into their bladders. Of those with previously uninjured bladders 12% developed tumours, whereas 54% of those with injured bladders developed tumours.

Whilst it is generally agreed that many patients have multifocal disease, with a generally unstable urothelium, the natural conclusion from these studies is that the urologist should consider not only the local destructive effect of any chosen therapeutic method but also its wider significance in terms of release of viable cells and surface injury elsewhere in the bladder.

Results of YAG Laser Treatment

So what evidence is there for improvement in treatment of superficial transitional cell cancer by YAG laser therapy? In particular, does it reduce tumour recurrence rates? Hofstetter has published a large series of reports detailing his group's experience with the YAG laser. Certainly the credit for the early experimental work and clinical application of the YAG laser must go to this group. In particular they laid down the therapeutic guidelines that most urologists have followed since. Hofstetter described local recurrence rates after YAG laser coagulation of 1.5% (Hofstetter and Frank 1980). His group has subsequently produced an impressive series of reports describing the treatment of large numbers of patients; however, relatively few patients have been reported as part of a prospective study, and of these the randomisation into four groups is such that statistical significance is unlikely without much larger numbers (Hofstetter 1986).

Staehler et al. (1985), in a study of 150 patients, described local recurrence rates of 5% in 60 patients with full follow-up. Staehler et al. studied patients with largely superficial disease (as far as they could determine) and 60% were treated with laser coagulation 4 days after TURB of protuberant, exophytic disease. The other 40% had laser treatment alone. However, recurrence rates elsewhere in the untreated areas of the bladder were 57%.

True local recurrence rates for other modalities are difficult to determine. An examination of the data in the papers previously referred to suggests local recurrence rates of between 30% and 50% with standard (non-laser) treatment (though many urologists would suggest this conflicts with their clinical impression of recurrence rates).

Many other groups in Europe, the USA and Japan have reported their experience following YAG laser coagulation of tumours. Malloy (1986) reported a 37% recurrence rate in 76 patients with superficial disease treated mainly as outpatients and with a 2-year follow-up period; Smith (1986a) described a 6% recurrence rate in the treatment site and 35% elsewhere in the bladder in 93 patients with superficial disease; and Shanberg et al. (1987) reported an 18% recurrence rate in 28 patients with T_1 disease.

Beisland et al. (1985) described their results in 100 consecutive patients, 53 of whom had new tumours and 47 recurrent tumours. Recurrences were carefully mapped in an attempt to separate those in the treated area from those occurring further afield. Patients underwent coagulation either by diathermy or YAG laser if tumours were small (less than 6 mm diameter) or TURB with or without YAG coagulation 2 weeks later if tumours were larger than 6 mm. Beisland et al. claimed a local recurrence rate of 7% after laser treatment at 3 months after treatment; in comparison 21% of patients developed a new occurrence of tumour in non-irradiated areas of the bladder over the same follow-up period.

These appear rather high rates at 3 months but were related to early treatments. The tumour development rate fell markedly on longer follow-up of later patients, so that, as the authors acknowledge, there may have been a "learning curve" effect initially. There was no difference in recurrence rates between patients who had been electroresected and subsequently laser irradiated and those who had been laser irradiated only. Arkell and Randall's (1988) first 12 patients underwent the successful coagulation of 54 of 55 original tumours with one recurrence in the treatment site, but 6 (50%) went on to develop further tumours elsewhere in the bladder.

Perhaps the best study available comes in a subsequent report from the Oslo group comparing local recurrence after YAG treatment with that following traditional electroresection and coagulation (TURB) (Beisland and Seland 1986). In this prospective randomised study 122 patients received either transurethral resection or laser treatment if small superficial T_a/T_1 tumours were found (less than 6 mm in diameter). Patients found to have larger though still superficial (T_a/T_1) tumours underwent tumour resection. They were then randomised to receive either laser coagulation to the resected area 2 weeks later or no further treatment. Only small tumours were treated either *purely* by laser or purely by electrocoagulation or electroresection (if the tumour was sufficiently small it could be removed by one pass of the 6-mm resectoscope loop). The authors demonstrated a significant decrease in local recurrence rates ($P<0.001$) in patients treated with the laser (3/62) compared with those treated with electrosurgery (19/60).

This interesting and well-designed trial indicates that small tumours are effectively treated by existing techniques or by laser, there being no local recurrences at a follow-up of 2 years. For T_a/T_1 tumours larger than 6 mm in diameter there was a statistically significant difference between those treated by TURB followed by laser treatment (no recurrences) and those treated by TURB alone (38% recurrences). In T_2 tumours with a diameter larger than 6 mm there was a 20% recurrence rate after TURB plus laser compared with 60% (6/10) following TURB alone. Overall laser recurrences were 4.8% compared with 31.6% after TURB alone. Recurrence rates in areas of the bladder remote from the treated areas were very similar whether the patient had been treated by laser or electroresection and electrocautery (20% compared with 22%). However, since 70% of the laser group had undergone electrosurgery prior to laser ablation, the implication is that they had larger tumours.

These results do seem to suggest that cutting through (larger) tumours is associated with an increased risk of recurrence, but it is not yet clear whether this is related to the larger size of the original tumour – which has previously been identified as a risk factor predisposing to the development of recurrences (Heney et al. 1982) – or whether it is related to the liberation of viable cells that subsequently seed elsewhere.

The experienced laser urologist would intuitively suspect that the visibly less violent process of laser coagulation would release fewer malignant cells than diathermy electroresection or coagulation, and a recent experimental study appears to support this previously unconfirmed impression. See and Chapman (1987) explored whether there was any difference between the effects of the YAG laser and electrocautery in a laboratory situation by a series of experiments based on the major steps of tumour cell implantation. They found that electrocautery, including electroresection of the tumour model by a resectoscope, followed by diathermy of its base, resulted in 620% more viable cells being liberated compared with the cells liberated by YAG laser coagulation of the same experimental model.

See and Chapman's experimental model involved the use of 3-methyl-cholanthrene-induced transitional cell carcinoma passaged in syngeneic Fisher 344 rats. A 1.5-cm diameter tumour, previously implanted subcutaneously into the right hindquarter of the animal, was dissected free from overlying skin, and the hind limb with tumour in situ excised and transected along a plane through the middle of the tumour. This gave two identical halves of tumour attached to lower limb musculature. One half was then "resected" using a 28Fr resectoscope, and the other half coagulated with the YAG laser so that complete thermal coagulation was achieved (to cause equal depth of tumour necrosis). At the end of the ablation/resection a 100-ml aliquot of the resection fluid was obtained and the cell count performed. Electrosurgery liberated 620% more viable cells and 729% more cells in total than laser ablation of an identical lesion. Adherence to the surfaces was also found to increase as a function of the concentration of cells present in the bathing medium.

This increase in the release of cells, if similarly produced in man, would be likely to increase the chance of successful tumour implantation and recurrence and may be expected to contribute to differences in recurrence rates after laser treatment. Experimental studies of tumour cell transplantation kinetics and other systems have demonstrated that the incidence of tumour growth is a direct function of initial tumour burden – in effect, of initial inoculum size (Porter et al. 1973).

See and Chapman's (1987) other studies of quantitative and qualitative cellular adherence of an equal number of cells to surfaces previously injured either by laser or by electroresection showed no significant differences between the two methods of coagulation.

There appears to be agreement in the literature that large, exophytic tumours require prior debulking by TURB. This is certainly our view. In addition TURB is still essential as part of the full staging of the patient's first tumour. Thus two suggested advantages of using the YAG laser – that fewer cells are liberated and that lymphatic coagulation may occur earlier – are going to be lost if the tumour has already been disrupted and disseminated by the electrosurgical process. Or at least the advantage has been lost in terms of a reduction of implantation possibilities in sites remote from the tumour; implantation within the tumour site may still be lower, as would appear to be borne out by the quoted local recurrence rates following laser coagulation.

Conclusion: Superficial Bladder Cancer

There is a small body of evidence suggesting that local tumour recurrence rates for superficial disease are indeed reduced by laser treatment. Recurrence rates elsewhere in the untreated areas are not obviously altered, and if this is due to a field change within the urothelium this is not surprising. Experimental evidence would seem to point to a reduced release of viable cells, particularly when laser coagulation was used alone rather than following TURB. However clinical evidence of any advantage resulting from this is as yet limited and in the small number of reports so far the recurrence rates in untreated areas appear to be similar whatever treatment method is used for the initial tumour. Outpatient treatment with minimal or no anaesthesia may prove a cost effective treatment option for those patients with superficial, well differentiated recurrences of their bladder tumour.

The Neodymium-YAG Laser in the Treatment of Muscle Invasive Bladder Cancer

In the case of invasive bladder cancer there is the prospect that in selected patients the deep thermal effects possible with the YAG laser might be as effective as radiotherapy or cystectomy; alternatively in those in whom cure is not possible, significant palliation may be achieved with minimum morbidity. We will examine the evidence for these claims.

The YAG laser produces a characteristically different pattern of coagulation from electrical energy even though it is still a thermal effect (Figs. 3.1 and 3.2). Diathermy current passes through tissue according to its electrical resistance. In a heterogeneous layered structure such as the bladder the coagulating current may spread out unevenly and conduct preferentially along paths of low resistance such as blood vessels. However, this spread is less marked and more focal if the diathermy energy is applied with coaptive pressure to the layers of the bladder wall. Laser energy, in contrast, generally produces a more confined, well demarcated area of coagulation, the depth of which relates to the applied energy. In the laboratory at least, a consistent transmural injury can be obtained without excessive forward scattering which could damage adjacent bowel. This sort of controlled lesion cannot reliably be produced by diathermy. Full-thickness resection and cautery has been advocated for the endoscopic control of muscle-invading tumour, but it is unlikely to become the accepted management without adjuvant therapy, especially chemotherapy (Hall et al. 1984).

Results of Conventional Treatment

Present routine treatment of localised bladder tumours which are invading muscle consists of cystectomy with urinary diversion or radiotherapy, either alone or in combination. A recent series of 182 patients with T_2 or T_3 bladder cancer showed an overall corrected 5-year survival rate of 40% following radical radiotherapy as the primary treatment, with salvage cystectomy for those (18%) who failed to respond, or who subsequently relapsed (Jenkins et al. 1988). Radiotherapy prior to radical cystectomy offers the potential of reducing pelvic recurrence and many older series showed the benefit from this combination. Skinner and Lieskovsky (1984) reported a series containing 197 patients with T_2 or T_3 cancer 97 of whom had radical surgery alone, the others preoperative adjuvant radiotherapy as well. There was no significant difference between the two groups, which both had a disease-free actuarial 5-year survival rate of about 50% pT_2 and pT_{3a}, 64%; pT_{3a} and pT_{3b}, 44%).

Results of YAG Laser Treatment

The three reported series of YAG-treated patients with invasive cancer for which there is adequate information about stage and treatment parameters involve quite small numbers of patients (Beisland and Seland 1986; Smith 1986b; McPhee et al. 1988). In addition, as with many trials of "new" treatments, they tend to consist largely of patients who are either unfit for or who refuse conventional treatment.

Beisland and Seland's (1986) prospective randomised trial included 25 patients with T_2 tumours, 15 of whom had laser treatment after TURB and 10 who had TURB only. After 4 years all were still alive, with 12 (80%) of the laser group free from recurrence in the treated area compared with only 4 (40%) in the TURB-only group. Recurrence of superficial disease elsewhere in the bladder was similar in both groups at around 20%. These results compare with local recurrences after treatment of superficial cancer of none out of 47 in the laser group and 13 out of 50 (26%) in the TURB-only group. Smith (1986b) reported 21 patients with muscle invasive tumour, 15 of whom had T_2 or T_3 tumours. Of these, 8 (53%) were disease-free at a mean follow-up of 1 year. Not surprisingly results were better in less advanced disease. Four of 5 patients with T_2 tumours were clear at 1 year, as were 3 of 6 with clinical stage T_{3a} (although 1 developed distant metastases), but only 1 of 4 T_{3b} patients was clear of local tumour. The 2 clinically T_{3a} patients without metastases were later staged P_{3b} after cystectomy. Six patients with bulky T_4 disease all seemed to be symptomatically improved after palliative laser treatment. One delayed perforation of the sigmoid colon was seen but there was no small bowel damage.

McPhee et al. (1988) treated 32 patients with a higher laser power (50–80 W) but used a diffusing tip to increase spot size; the power density was therefore probably less than that used by other groups. There was one post-operative death (cardiac) but no instance of bowel perforation. Crude survival for T_2 and T_3 tumours was 58% (50% disease-free) at follow-up after between 4 months and 6 years. Once again results were good for T_2 tumours, with no local recurrence in 12 patients after 6–72 months of follow-up, though 40% developed T_1 recurrences elsewhere in the bladder. Four of 7 patients with T_{3a} cancer had a recurrence and 3 died (only 1 with cancer). All 7 patients with T_{3b} tumours died, 1 post-operatively and the other 6 with recurrences. All 6 who received palliation for T_4 tumours also died.

The risk of clinical understaging, especially of T_{3b} tumours, is clearly present and laser therapy would not be expected to cure a tumour which had spread outside the bladder wall. Nevertheless effective local control of about 80% of T_2 tumours seems possible with minimal morbidity in patients who are largely unfit for radical surgery. One worrying feature is that re-epithelialisation may cover viable nests of tumour cells deep in the bladder wall and compromise detection until sizeable extravesical recurrence has occurred.

A major problem is the inability to guarantee a consistent full-thickness necrosis in the clinical setting despite what seems achievable experimentally. One possible solution, though it would increase morbidity, might be to irradiate appropriately situated tumours from both the mucosal and serosal aspects, or at least to monitor the serosal temperature during treatment. In a series of patients undergoing endoscopic laser coagulation prior to cystectomy we were able to guarantee full-thickness coagulation, monitoring the effects of endoscopic laser coagulation on the serosal surface of the bladder either visually or by thermometry (Fig. 3.3). Alternatively we applied laser energy to both the mucosal aspect (endoscopically) and the serosal surface (exposed at operation). Much higher total energies were required to achieve visible serosal effects than would have been expected from the guidelines suggested by the German laser pioneers.

Unfortunately these acute studies all suffer from the disadvantage that a much lower energy might just as successfully achieve full-thickness coagulation if the specimen or subject were allowed 3–4 days to develop the full tissue response to the laser injury.

Until more accurate dosimetry is possible it is prudent to select patients carefully for laser treatment; those with either T_2 tumours or those with T_{3a} cancer who are unfit for or refuse cystectomy are suitable. It seems possible that when large numbers of patients have been treated by YAG laser therapy after TURB, the results in T_2 bladder cancer might bear comparison with the best results after radical radiotherapy or surgery, with a fraction of the morbidity that these conventional treatments involve.

Conclusion: Invasive Bladder Cancer

For muscle-invading tumours laser treatment is only indicated, at present, in carefully selected patients who are either not candidates for radical treatment because of age or distant metastatic disease, or who categorically refuse bladder

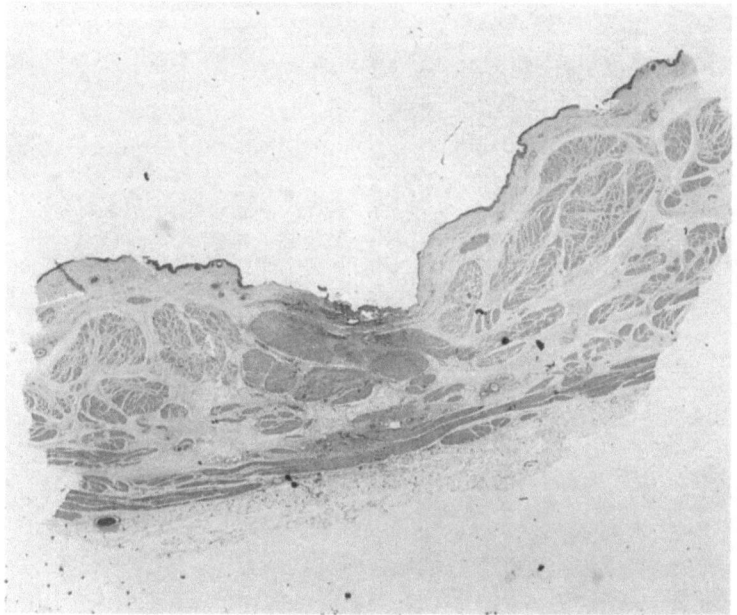

Fig. 3.3. Full thickness YAG laser coagulation of human bladder (6 mm thick and coagulated prior to cystectomy).

removal or radiotherapy. It can also be used as palliative therapy in an attempt to debulk large tumours with extravesical extension and side wall fixation, and particularly as a haemostatic treatment for troublesome and resistant haemorrhage from incurable tumours. Laser therapy for invasive bladder tumours is still in its infancy and at the present time laser treatment can only be realistically applied to superficial bladder tumours.

Urethral Tumours

Urethral transitional cell carcinoma in association with extensive disease of the bladder is clearly best treated by cystourethrectomy. The position is not so clear when the bladder is either devoid of tumour or, more commonly, the tumour present in the bladder is minimal and can be regarded as endoscopically controllable. In these circumstances some form of local therapy for the urethral tumours is desirable unless or until the surgeon feels that cystourethrectomy is necessary.

The urethra is unforgiving of most treatments and exhibits a tendency to cicatrisation and stricture formation, particularly after high-frequency electrocoagulation (Mauermayer 1983). Topical preparations of chemotherapeutic agents may also lead to stricturing as well as meatitis, dysuria and scrotal irritation (Sand et al. 1987). In the absence of an obvious "ideal" treatment we felt that the use of the YAG laser energy in the urethra might represent a possible alternative treatment for extensive urethral transitional cell tumour. We have assessed the YAG laser in the management of patients with multiple urethral

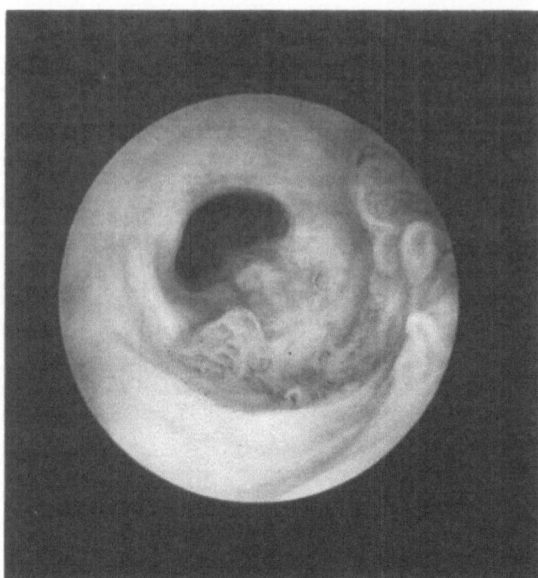

Fig. 3.4. Multiple urethral tumours.

tumours in whom traditional treatments had failed or were thought likely to cause extensive urethral damage due to the widespread nature of the tumours (Fig. 3.4).

Methods

Six patients with extensive urethral transitional cell tumours were treated. In 5 the previous pathological diagnosis was confirmed. In one man of 39 with very extensive papillary growths and areas of flat, abnormal epithelium in the urethra, further pathological review involving viral DNA gene probing suggested a viral aetiology, the transitional epithelium displaying hyperplasia, squamous metaplasia and dysplasia with vacuolated cytoplasm. In each case tumour appeared to be superficial, was impalpable in the urethra and on biopsy was G_1 or G_2 in tumour grading.

After urethrocystoscopy with mapping and biopsy of urethral lesions, a "test treatment" was performed on lesions within a 1-cm long circumferential strip of mid-penile urethra using the YAG laser (Living Technology Fiberlase 100) at a power of 20 W for short pulses (1–2 seconds) until the target tissue shrank and became a uniformly white colour representing coagulation of tissue proteins (Fig. 3.5, opposite p.56). The laser beam was conducted along a 600-μm diameter quartz glass fibre passed down the instrument channel of a cystoscope or more usually a 20Ch urethrotome.

Patients with transitional cell tumours of the prostatic urethra are known to be at risk of invasion and metastatic spread and are best treated by radical clearance; consequently laser treatment was not directed at tumours situated in the prostatic urethra.

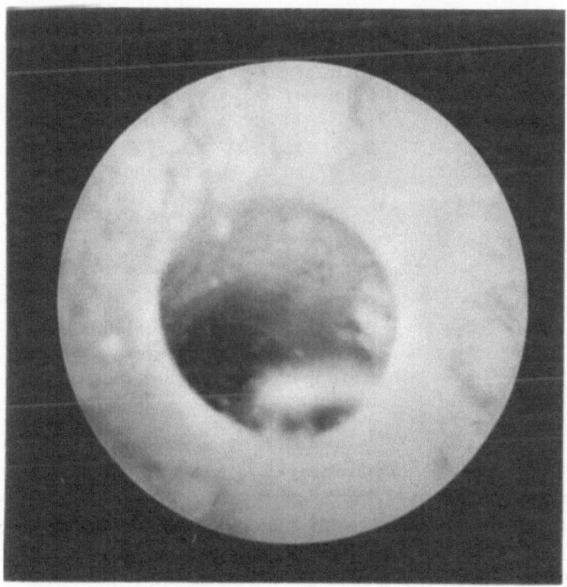

Fig. 3.6. Focal urethral stricture following laser coagulation of mass of urethral tumour.

Endoscopy was repeated 6 weeks later to assess the urethral response to laser coagulation and particularly to see whether stricture formation had occurred. If the urethral appearances were satisfactory as much tumour as possible was treated at 6-weekly intervals, followed by check endoscopy at 3 months and 6 months following completion of treatment.

In one patient with a relatively large mass of tumour in his mid-penile urethra which required a large energy application we found a discrete circumferential stricture which was easily managed by one dilatation at the time of check endoscopy (Fig. 3.6). Details of the first 4 patients with significant follow-up are shown in Table 3.1.

Discussion and Conclusion

YAG laser energy effectively coagulates scattered small papillary tumours of the urethra with little or no risk of stricturing even when multiple areas require coagulation. The treatment of large focal masses of tumour can lead to superficial stricturing which does not appear to extend deep into the urethral wall and which is readily dilated. Such masses of urethral tumour would previously have been amenable only to urethrectomy.

One of our patients, previously treated with radiotherapy, whose urethral tumours had been almost entirely cleared with laser therapy, was awaiting cystectomy on account of recurrent bladder and prostatic urethral tumour when he rapidly developed abnormal liver function tests followed by clinical evidence of metastatic liver disease within the space of 3 months.

Tumours within the glandular urethra and fossa navicularis are relatively difficult to manage with existing cystoscopes due to the poor visualisation in

Table 3.1. Results of YAG laser treatment of tumours occupying the whole length of the urethra

Patient no. (age)	No. treatments	Total energy (J)	Flow rate (ml/s)	Stricture	Tumours cleared	Urethral follow-up	Residual tumour elsewhere
1 (79)	2	3 400	–	No	Yes	Clear (except FN)[a]	Prostatic urethra and within FN
2 (76)	3	16 500	22	No	Yes	Clear	No
3 (31)	4	5 200	40	No	Yes	Clear	No
4 (74)[b]	2	9 300	–	Yes, dilated	No	Small area of persistent mid-penile tumour and a mass of prostatic urethral tumour (previously resected)	Recurrent p_{1b} G_2 tumour in bladder and prostatic urethra following radiotherapy[c]

[a]Tumours within the FN (fossa navicularis) are difficult to get adequate access to and tend to be relatively undertreated.
[b]This patient developed metastatic disease whilst awaiting cystectomy.
[c]Prostatic urethral and bladder tumours *not* treated by laser in this series.

this part of the terminal urethra. We have found the visual urethrotome a better but not ideal instrument for examination and treatment in this region. To overcome this difficulty a purpose-designed "meatoscope" is invaluable and a suitable prototype instrument is now being used to inspect and treat this area. This is described in Chap. 5 and illustrated in Fig. 5.6.

If a YAG laser is available it may be used in an attempt to maintain endoscopic control of scattered papillary urethral tumours. The endoscopic use of the YAG laser was an effective and safe treatment, particularly for multiple, superficial papillary tumours of the urethra.

Tumours of the Ureter and Pelvicaliceal System

Our clinical studies of the endoscopic use of the YAG laser for the treatment of bladder tumours in comparison with traditional electroresection suggested no very obvious immediate advantages that had not been fully explored elsewhere. This led us to consider treating conditions where there were particular treatment difficulties and where the use of the YAG laser appeared to offer advantages over existing treatment methods. Transitional cell tumours of the urethra and upper urinary tract appeared to be such problems.

Current treatment of transitional cell cancers of the ureter and pelvicaliceal system usually involves nephro-ureterectomy. However, the place of more conservative treatment is increasingly being considered (Reitelman et al. 1987). Whilst this generally means local resection for ureteric tumours or local resection of pelvicaliceal tumours exposed at open operation it must increas-

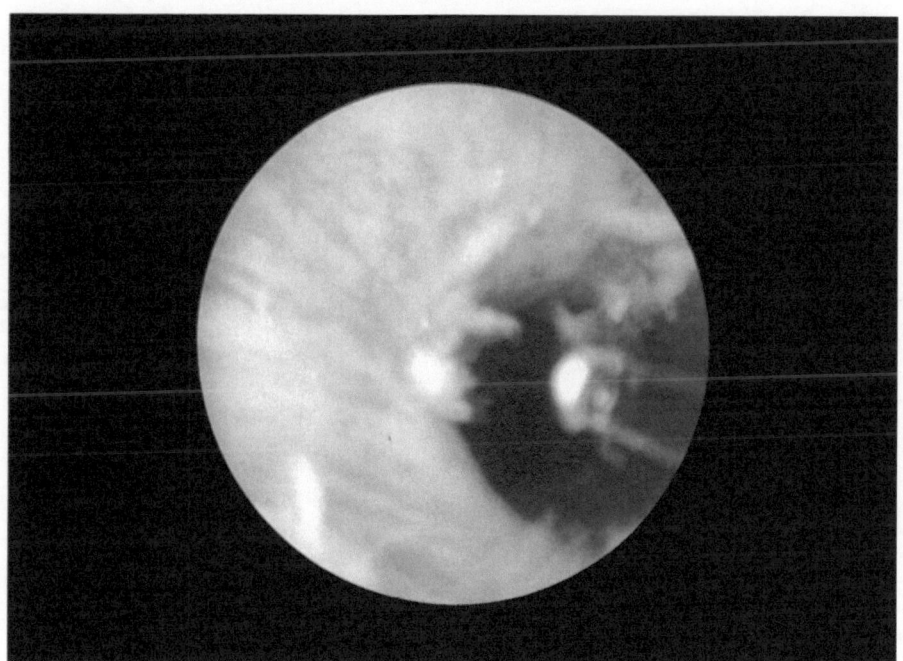

Fig. 3.5. YAG laser fibre coagulating tumours in urethra.

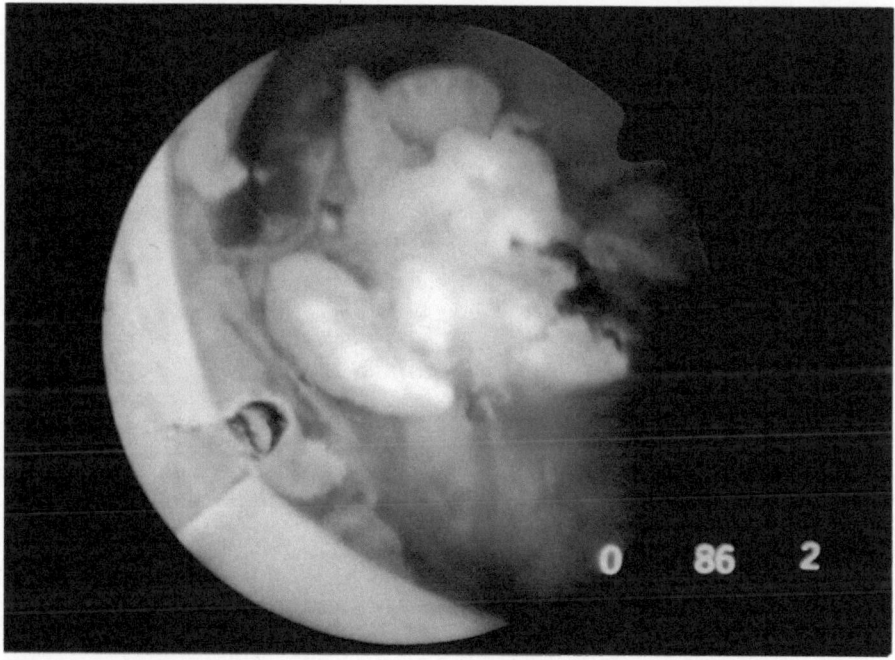

Fig. 3.7. Tumour in an upper pole calyx in a solitary kidney undergoing endoscopic laser coagulation (successful palliative treatment for haemorrhage).

ingly be considered whether a totally endoscopic method of treatment would be as good.

The challenge is to develop methods whereby superficial, relatively low-grade tumours of the ureter and pelvicaliceal system can be treated in an endoscopic manner in the way that tumours of the same grade and stage which occur in the bladder are treated. The rapid developments in the endoscopic armamentarium for upper tract endoscopy appear to make that possibility more realistic. All urologists will be aware of the developments in endoscopic treatment of upper tract stone disease and it will come as no surprise to hear that where an endoscope has been passed then a laser fibre is sure to follow!

Historical Background

Watson's pioneering work with the pulse dye laser for ureteric stone destruction (Watson and Wickham 1986) was the real beginning of the upper tract laser era, although in 1984 Hofstetter had described ureteroscopic laser coagulation of ureteric tumours with no complications and no post-laser strictures. Smith (1987) described the laser treatment of four tumours in the intramural ureter; he found treatment at this site to be particularly safe and to carry a much reduced risk of perforation due to the thickness of the urinary bladder. Malloy (1985) has described the use of the YAG laser for coagulation of tumours within the upper collecting system through an open pyelotomy incision, care being taken to avoid spillage of cells into the open wound. In our view, this has no advantages over a percutaneous technique and may well be more prone to the risks of seeding.

The same reasons for the use of the laser as an energy source for stone destruction also apply to tumour destruction in the upper urinary tract and particularly to ureteric tumours. Although ureteroscopes have improved in quality and are much reduced in size (which reduces the damage to the ureter by the passage of the endoscope itself) there remains the problem of how to get an adequate supply of energy to achieve the desired therapeutic effect once endoscopic access has been gained. The principal advantage of the laser, of course, is that relatively large amounts of energy can be passed down small-calibre transmitting fibres, and indeed using the YAG laser these same small fibres can allow relatively deep and reliable coagulation at the target site. Once again the laser is being used partly because it may be a more effective coagulator but perhaps more importantly because it can be used relatively easily in the ureter.

Such endoscopic local treatment of a transitional cell carcinoma of the upper tract is at present only indicated when traditional treatment is unsuitable. Patients with solitary kidneys, bilateral ureteric or renal tumours, or patients who are poor operative risks (or indeed who refuse a more radical procedure) can be considered. However, at present the technique should be used only by those who have both laser and upper tract endoscopic experience and who are prepared to deal with any complications which might ensue. It is our hope and expectation that with increasing experience and further technological developments the ultimate goal of the endoscopic management of upper tract tumours will be realised.

Ureteric Tumours

In many ways ureteric tumours are a more straightforward problem for the upper tract laser endoscopist than intrarenal tumours. Ureteric tumours can be approached with the ureteroscope to allow a direct biopsy and endoscopic assessment. Alternatively cytological brushings can be performed from the bladder thereby avoiding one diagnostic ureteroscopy. We use an 11.5Fr Wolf ureteroscope or the 9.5Fr Storz ureteroscope with the movable eyepiece. The ureteric orifice frequently will not require dilatation prior to using the smaller instruments now available, particularly if these are introduced with a degree of hydrostatic dilatation of the orifice. The Storz Ureteromat is suitable for this and includes sensitive safety features such as feedback pressure monitoring which cuts off the irrigation if certain pressure parameters within the ureter are exceeded; with care less sophisticated pressure infusion devices can be used.

For therapeutic ureteroscopy ureteric lesions can be approached either retrograde from below or anterograde through a percutaneous puncture of the kidney. A flexible ureteroscope is an attractive option when introduced through a percutaneous nephrostomy tract and down the ureter.

There is little literature defining appropriate power settings for treating lesions of the ureter or renal pelvicaliceal system. However, given a ureteric wall thickness of only 1–1.5 mm, our experimental and subsequent clinical studies have dictated a reduction of power from that used in the bladder to 15–20 W, and we limit application in one area to no longer than approximately 2 seconds. Smith (1983) found that higher powers (60 W) for shorter periods (0.5 seconds) were less likely to perforate the dog ureter than were the parameters we use. Excessive photoradiation causes carbonisation of the tumour and possibly perforation of the ureteric wall. In practice, though, the ureter is usually coagulated by firing the laser at the tumour site relatively obliquely, thereby reducing the power density at the laser impact site and acting as a safety valve.

Whenever extensive areas are coagulated or where there is any doubt about the patency of the ureteric wall – or indeed where access to the site of the ureteric tumour has been difficult – then a double-J ureteric stent should be left in place for approximately 4 weeks to combat post-operative ureteric oedema. The stent can be removed by flexible or rigid cystoscopy under local anaesthetic and the region examined with the ureteroscope when the inflammatory response to treatment and to the presence of the stent has settled, i.e. at about 3 months.

Clinical studies have been sparse and mainly show the technical feasibility of this approach rather than confirming an advantage over other forms of local treatment. In practice many experienced laser users who have an interest in upper tract endoscopy have applied the YAG laser in this way. Shanberg has a series of 10 patients with lower ureteric tumours of low grade (G_1/G_2) whom he has treated with 20–25-W power settings and 2-second pulses. He advises the use of a mixture of lignocaine (lidocaine) gel injected up the ureter as a combination of lubricant and antispasmodic (A. Shanberg, personal communication 1989).

Pelvicaliceal Tumours

The situation is more difficult for tumours of the pelvicaliceal system and particularly for tumours of the renal pelvis. The renal pelvis is as thin as the ureter and tumours within it may be situated in such a position that adequate laser coagulation might put at risk adjacent structures such as the renal vessels and the gut. Obviously in other parts of the pelvis adequate coagulation would be safer. However, in a series of reports on the endoscopic treatment of renal pelvic tumours using the resectoscope an incidence of perforation has been found to be acceptable (Woodhouse et al. 1986), so it is likely that laser coagulation will be as safe.

For tumours situated in the caliceal system the much greater volume of tissue underlying the tumour greatly reduces the risks of onward transmission of the laser energy beyond the tumour.

Upper tract renal pelvicaliceal tumours should be assessed radiologically and cytologically as are any other tumours of the upper urinary tract. Access to them is in practice much more reasonable through a percutaneous track, though the risks of seeding have to be considered. If only low-grade tumours are chosen for this localised treatment - which is in our view the only appropriate group for this treatment - then the risks of implantation are low. The risks of implantation can be further reduced by the use of an iridium wire inserted along the percutaneous track as described by Woodhouse et al. (1986).

With future developments, particularly of flexible ureteronephroscopes, the distinct possibility arises of access to all parts of the pelvicaliceal system by passage of the flexible ureteroscope from the bladder. This is still some way off though; it should also be remembered that repeated regular endoscopic access is necessary following such treatment, without which a single endoscopic treatment may not advance treatment significantly.

We have a series of patients in whom pelvicaliceal tumours have been treated for palliative reasons - usually repeated haemorrhage from tumours in patients with disseminated disease or who are unfit for other, more aggressive therapy. We have been impressed by the palliative effects achieved in these patients. Such a case is illustrated in Fig. 3.7 (opposite p.56, where a caliceal tumour in a solitary kidney can be seen undergoing laser coagulation.

References

Bladder

Anon (1986) Superficial bladder cancer: drugs or diathermy? Lancet i:479–480
Arkell DG, Randall J (1988) Installation and use of a neodymium YAG laser in a urological department. Br J Urol 62:398–404
Beisland HO, Seland P (1986) A prospective randomized study on neodymium-YAG laser irradiation versus TUR in the treatment of urinary bladder cancer. Scand J Urol Nephrol 20:209–212
Beisland HO, Sander S, Fossberg E (1985) Nd YAG laser irradiation of urinary bladder tumours. Urology 25:559–563

Benson RC (1988) Treatment of bladder cancer with haematoporphyrin derivative and laser light. Urology [Suppl] 31:13-17

Bown SG, Salmon PR, Storey DW, Calder BM, Kelly DF, Adams N, Pearson H, Weaver BMQ (1980) Nd YAG laser photocoagulation in the dog stomach. Gut 21:818-825

Boyd PJR, Burnand KG (1974) Site of bladder tumour recurrence. Lancet ii:1290-1292

Cutler SJ, Heney NM, Friedell GH (1982) Longitudinal study of patients with bladder cancer: factors associated with disease recurrence and progression. In: Bonney WW, Prout GR (eds) Bladder cancer. Williams and Wilkins, Baltimore, pp 35-46 (AUA monograph, vol 1)

Flannigan GM, Gelister JSK, Noble JG, Milroy EJG (1988) Rigid versus flexible cystoscopy: a controlled trial of patient tolerance. Br J Urol 62:537-540

Hall RR, Newling DWW, Ramsden PD, Richards B, Robinson MRG, Smith PH (1984) Treatment of invasive bladder cancer by local resection and high dose methotrexate. Br J Urol 56:668-672

Heney NM, Nocks BN, Daly JJ, Prout GR, Newall JB, Griffin PP, Perrone TL, Szyfelbein WA (1982) T_a and T_1 bladder cancer: location, recurrence and progression. Br J Urol 54:152-157

Hofstetter A (1986) Treatment of urological tumors by neodymium-YAG laser. Eur Urol 12 [Suppl]:21-24

Hofstetter AG (1987) Neodymium:YAG laser treatment of bladder tumours. J Endourology 1:115-117

Hofstetter A, Frank F (1980) The Nd YAG laser in urology. Editions "Roche", Hoffman La Roche, Basle, Switzerland

Jenkins BJ, Caulfield MJ, Fowler CG, Badenoch DF, Tiptaft RC, Paris AMI, Hope-Stone HF, Oliver RT, Blandy JP (1988) Reappraisal of the role of radical radiotherapy and salvage cystectomy in the treatment of invasive (T_2/T_3) bladder cancer. Br J Urol 62:343-346

Malloy TR (1986) Neodymium:YAG laser in transitional cell cancer of the bladder with emphasis on outpatient potential. Eur Urol 12 [Suppl]:25-27

McPhee MS, Arnfield MR, Tulip J, Lakey WH (1988) Neodymium:YAG laser therapy for infiltrating bladder cancer. J Urol 140:44-46

Mulvaney WP, Beck CW (1968) The laser beam in urology. J Urol 99:112-115

Mussiggang H, Katsaros W (1971) A study of the possibilities of laser surgery. Int Urol Nephrol 3:229-243

Nath G, Gorisch W, Kiefhaber P (1973) First laser endoscopy via a fibreoptic transmission system. Endoscopy 5:208-213

Page BH, Levison VB, Curwen MP (1978) The site of recurrence of non-infiltrating bladder tumours. Br J Urol 50:237-242

Parsons RL, Campbell JL, Thomley MW, Butt CG, Gordon TE (1966) The effect of the laser on dog bladders: a preliminary report. J Urol 95:716-717

Pensel J, Hofstetter A, Frank F, Keiditsch E, Rothenberger K (1981) Temporal and spatial temperature profile of the bladder serosa in intravesical Neodymium YAG laser irradiation. Eur Urol 7:298-303

Pope AJ, McNicholas TA (1989) Morphological effects of the Nd:YAG laser compared to electrocautery on the bladder. Presentation to the British Association of Urological Surgeons, Jersey, 21 June 1989

Porter EH, Hewit HB, Blake ER (1973) The transplantation kinetics of tumour cells. Br J Cancer 27:55-62

Schaeffer AJ (1986) Use of the CO_2 laser in urology. Urol Clin N Am 13:393-404

See WA, Chapman WA (1987) Tumour cell implantation following neodymium:YAG bladder injury: a comparison to electrocautery injury. J Urol 137:1266-1269

Shanberg AM, Baghdassarian R, Tansey LA (1987) Use of the Nd YAG laser in treatment of bladder cancer. Urology 24:26-30

Skinner DG, Lieskovsky G (1984) Contemporary cystectomy with pelvic node dissection compared to preoperative radiation therapy plus cystectomy in management of invasive bladder cancer. J Urol 131:1069-1072

Smith JA Jr (1986a) Endoscopic applications of laser energy. Urol Clin N Am 13:405-419

Smith JA Jr (1986b) Treatment of invasive bladder cancer with neodymium:YAG laser. J Urol 135:55-57

Smith JA Jr, Dixon J (1984) Argon laser phototherapy of superficial transitional cell carcinoma of the bladder. J Urol 131:655-656

Smith JA, Landau S (1989) Neodymium YAG laser specifications for safe intravesical therapy. J Urol 141:1238-1239

Soloway MS, Masters S (1980) Urothelial susceptibility to tumour cell implantation: influence of cauterization. Cancer 46:1158-1163

Staehler G. Hofstetter A (1979) Transurethral laser irradiation of urinary bladder tumours. Eur Urol 5:64–69

Staehler G. Hofstetter A. Gorisch W. Keiditsch E. Mussiggang H (1976) Endoscopy in experimental urology using an argon laser beam. Endoscopy 8:1–4

Staehler G. Halldorsson T. Langerholc J. Bilgram R (1981) Endoscopic applications of the Nd:YAG and CO_2 lasers: bladder and kidney. Lasers Surg Med 6:353–363

Staehler G. Chaussy C. Jocham D. Schmiedt E (1985) The use of Nd YAG laser in urology: indication, technique and critical assessment. J Urol 134:1155–1160

Stein BS (1986) Urologic dosimetry studies with the Nd:YAG and CO_2 lasers: bladder and kidney. Lasers Surg Med 6:353–363

Union Internationale Contre le Cancer (UICC) (1978) TNM classification of malignant tumours. 3rd end. International Union Against Cancer. Geneva

Weldon TE. Soloway MS (1975) Susceptibility of urothelium to cellular implantation. Urology 5:824–827

Zimmerman I. Stern J. Frank F. Keiditsch E. Hofstetter A (1984) Interception of lymphatic drainage by Nd:YAG laser irradiation in rat urinary bladder. Lasers Surg Med 4:167–172

Urethra

Mauermayer W (1983) Endoscopic surgery for urethral tumours. In: Transurethral surgery. Springer. Berlin Heidelberg New York. p 389

Sand PK. Shen W. Bowen LW. Ostergard DR (1987) Cryotherapy for the treatment of proximal urethral condylomata acuminata. J Urol 137:874–876

Ureter and Pelvicaliceal System

Hofstetter A (1984) Laser application for destroying ureteral tumours. Lasers Surg Med 3:152

Malloy TR (1985) Laser treatment of the ureter and upper collecting system. In: Smith JA (ed) Lasers in urologic surgery. Year Book Medical Publishers. Chicago. p 87

Reitelman C. Sawczuk IS. Olsson CA. Puchner PJ. Benson MC (1987) Prognostic variables in patients with transitional cell carcinoma of the renal pelvis and proximal ureter. J Urol 138:1144–1145

Smith JA (1983) Nd YAG laser photoradiation of canine ureters: an analysis of penetration depth and subsequent healing. Surg Forum 34:696–697

Smith JA (1987) Application of laser energy in urologic surgery. In: De Vere White RW. Palmer JM (eds) New techiques in urology. Futura Publishing. New York. p 179

Watson GM. Wickham JEA (1986) Initial experience with a pulse dye laser for ureteric calculi. Lancet i:1357–1358

Woodhouse CRJ. Kellett MJ. Bloom HJG (1986) Percutaneous renal surgery and local radiotherapy in the management of renal pelvic transitional cell carcinoma. Br J Urol 58:245–249

Chapter 4

Laser Treatment of Urological Tumours 2: Carcinoma of the Prostate and Penis

T. A. McNicholas

Carcinoma of the Prostate

Introduction

Carcinoma of the prostate is the commonest urological cancer and is the fifth commonest malignant tumour of males worldwide (Parkin et al. 1984). It remains one of the major challenges in urology. In the UK it characteristically presents to urologists at a late stage with extensive local disease and/or metastases (Chisholm and Habib 1981), though in much of Western Europe and North America approximately half the cases will be potentially curable with small-volume, localised disease.

Particular problems remain in the effective treatment of "early" prostatic cancer. Firstly, there is the fact that with increasing age the majority of prostate glands will exhibit some evidence of focal carcinoma of the prostate (Franks 1954). The incidence of incidental or latent carcinoma of the prostate appears high, whereas the clinical incidence of the disease, although an important cause of morbidity and death compared with other malignant processes, is lower than it should be if it is indeed the case that all these tumours will inevitably progress. Therefore it has appeared that many "early" cancers if found may not progress, and particularly in those presenting at an advanced age will not cause clinically significant problems. However, there remains the strong possibility that even small volumes of relatively low-grade tumour in a younger male may well lead, in the fullness of time, to clinically significant problems.

McNeal et al. (1986) have provided more information on this possibility in a study during which post-mortem specimens found to contain carcinoma of the prostate were examined to see whether tumour progression was related to tumour size or other features. They found 100 glands with evidence of adenocarcinoma among 436 males examined post-mortem. They measured the volume of the largest mass of tumour found in the gland (in many cases there was more than one area of tumour). In addition the histological grade was assessed according to the Gleason system (Gleason et al. 1974), and the presence, depth and extent of capsular invasion and involvement of the seminal vesicles was also recorded. The post-mortem studies showed that increase in tumour volume was strongly correlated with a progressive loss of differentiation, the presence and extent of capsular penetration and the likelihood of metastatic spread. Metastases were only found in association with a tumour volume above 4 ml and only 13% of cases of tumours were that big (80% of the tumours were smaller than 1.4 ml and 60% smaller than 0.46 ml).

When applied to the pathological findings in radical prostatectomy specimens from 38 males, metastatic disease to lymph nodes (found at staging lymphadenectomy) was associated with large volumes (above 4 ml) but the relationship was not statistically significant. Grade, though, was significantly related to both volume and metastatic disease.

From this study McNeal et al. concluded that tumours start small and well differentiated. As they grow they lose differentiation and acquire the capacity for metastasis, probably expressed largely in tumours above 1 ml in volume. The authors feel that carcinoma of the prostate does indeed follow a predictable course. The high incidence of adenocarcinoma in post-mortem studies ("latent carcinoma") without a high incidence of clinical signs or evidence of metastases can be explained by their finding that most of the tumours in the post-mortem series were below 1 ml in volume and could be expected to remain silent for a long time. The clinically undetected "latent cancers" reported from the post-mortem series are not, therefore, a separate disease entity but are in most cases recent developments (as a manifestation of the sharply rising age-specific incidence curve), and are too small to be detectable or to have achieved metastatic potential.

It follows that the presence of prostatic cancer in the younger male does put him at risk of disease progression, even if the extent of the tumour is apparently very small, purely by virtue of his longer time at risk.

Even the supposition that for many, especially the elderly, the development of prostatic adenocarcinoma may not be life threatening can be challenged. Adami et al. (1986) took advantage of the sophisticated population recording systems available in Sweden to study 44 300 cases of prostatic cancer recorded in the Swedish Cancer Registry between 1960 and 1978. They measured relative survival, defined as the difference between the observed rate of survival in the prostatic cancer group and the rate expected for the general population corresponding to the studied group. This measure therefore corresponds to the probability of *not* dying from prostatic cancer. They found that the relative survival after 5, 10 and 15 years was 51%, 34% and 24% respectively. There was an annual excess death rate of approximately 8% for the prostatic cancer group, rising to 10% for those above 74 years of age. The study supports the view that clinically diagnosed carcinoma of the prostate does not behave in "benign fashion" even at an advanced stage and does in fact significantly affect survival whenever diagnosed.

The challenge to the clinician is whether he can pick out those at particularly high risk of significant tumour development. A large number of prognostic factors have been examined in an attempt to define the risk of progression for any particular patient's tumour, including histological assessments of the grade of the tumour by either the Gleason scoring system (Gleason et al. 1974) or that described by Mostofi (Mostofi 1975). This has increasingly been shown to correlate with the likelihood of lymph node spread (Paulson 1980).

An encouraging finding of McNeal's report (1986) is that the features to which metastatic potential was related, i.e. volume, depth and extent of capsular invasion and seminal vesicle involvement, are all increasingly measurable or detectable, particularly with ultrasound. Flow cytometry may also have an increasing role to play (Fordham et al. 1986). Finally, serological tests in particular serum acid phosphatase and prostate specific antigen levels will, if elevated, suggest the presence of extraprostatic disease. Thus the possibility arises of increased accuracy of prognosis which may allow surgeons to focus curative therapy on younger males who can reliably be expected not to have developed metastatic spread already.

The utilisation of all these prognostic features may help in consideration of the clinical problem in the treatment of apparently localised prostatic cancer, i.e. the case of the relatively young male (below 65) with a histologically proven focus of tumour and no evidence of extraprostatic spread. Should this apparently localised tumour reveal, on pathological examination, features particularly on Gleason or Mostofi scoring that suggest a moderately or poorly differentiated tumour with an increased likelihood of local or distant progression, then an attempt at curative treatment appears to be indicated in the absence of evidence of distant spread.

Such a patient, if diagnosed after transurethral resection of the prostate (TURP), will be staged by the TNM system (UICC 1978) as either T_{0a} if 5% or less of the resected chips are positive for tumour on pathological examination (Ford et al. 1984) or T_{0b} if more than 5% of the chips are positive. This subclassification was first suggested by Jewett (1975), using the American classification notation of A_1 and A_2. It seems clear that those falling into the T_{0b} (A_2) group have a much more gloomy prognosis than the T_{0a} (A_1) group and indeed worse than T_1 disease (Cantrell et al. 1981; Sheldon et al. 1980; Beynon et al. 1983) and require more aggressive treatment.

However, the choice of a potentially curative treatment for early, apparently localised disease remains problematical. This is partly due to the difficulties inherent in trying to show a clear curative advantage for one modality over another in a condition with a prolonged and variable natural course. In addition the condition is perceived as affecting a relatively elderly male population and the morbidity of existing potentially curative treatment may be seen as excessive.

Both radical surgery and radical radiotherapy have significant complications and side effects. Radical surgery is frequently associated with impotence (85%–90%: Walsh and Jewett 1980) and incontinence (13%: Smith and Kelly 1984), although recent developments in methods of surgical removal of the gland, sparing the neurovascular bundles, have contributed to a reduction in the incidence of these serious complications (Walsh and Mostwin 1984). Radical radiotherapy commits the patient to a 6–8-week course of daily treatment, and even in the hands of the most experienced a significant complication rate of 10%–12% has been reported (Ray and Bagshaw 1975). Experience elsewhere in Europe and the UK has confirmed that severe side effects can be expected from radiotherapy in from 30% (Ritchie et al. 1985) to as high as 74% of cases (Lindholt and Hansen 1986). Incontinence is unusual but impotence is probably more common than has been realised, even though it occurs gradually (presumably as a result of radiation-induced vascular damage) rather than abruptly as after surgery. Goldstein et al. (1984) reported that 79% of their 19 potent patients closely followed up after definitive radiotherapy became irreversibly impotent at an average of 14 months after treatment and their investigations suggested a vascular aetiology due to damage to vessels within the radiation field.

Although results from long-term studies are not yet available, seed implantation appears to be associated with a disease-free survival lower than that after radical surgery or radiotherapy; however, complications are similarly reduced (Nag 1985). In our experience seed implantation techniques have been hampered by logistical problems related to the supply of the seeds, their cost and the complex arrangements required for their implantation (Carter et al. 1987).

Therefore an alternative approach to curative therapy that avoids the morbidity of radical surgery or radiotherapy would be of great benefit. Ideally, such treatment would be endoscopic rather than requiring major open surgery. It would be applicable to prostatic tumour within any part of the gland, would have an acceptable incidence of side effects, and particularly would have no adverse effects on potency or continence.

Endoscopic Laser Coagulation of the Prostate

In the early 1980s a novel technique was reported (Sander et al. 1982; Sander and Beisland 1984) that combined a radical resection of the prostate to remove the bulk of tissue and "debulk" the tumour, followed by photocoagulation of the remaining prostatic capsule with the neodymium yttrium aluminium garnet (YAG) laser in an attempt to sterilise any remaining cancer cells in the capsule. Their initial results were encouraging in terms of disease-free survivals and there were no instances of impotence or incontinence (Beisland and Sander 1986).

We adapted this technique in the light of our own experience in an attempt to determine whether the boundaries of endoscopic treatment for localised carcinoma of the prostate could be extended further (McNicholas et al. 1988a). Patients who appeared to have disease localised to the prostate and a normal bone scan were entered into a pilot trial. A detailed sexual history and an assessment of continence were recorded for each patient.

Ultrasound scanning was performed (a) on referral to the Prostate Unit, (b) under anaesthesia, (c) prior to the extended TURP, and (d) usually after extended transurethral resection of the prostate (when the image is often obscured by blood which causes a lot of acoustic echoes, so that repeated ultrasound assessment some weeks later is usually of more value). The ultrasound assessment was in any case repeated before laser treatment and of course in the period after treatment.

The Bruel and Kjaer 1850 ultrasound scanner was used with the relatively well known 5.5 or 7 megahertz (MHz) axial scanning transducer. This gives a series of cross-sectional slices or images through the prostate from posterior to

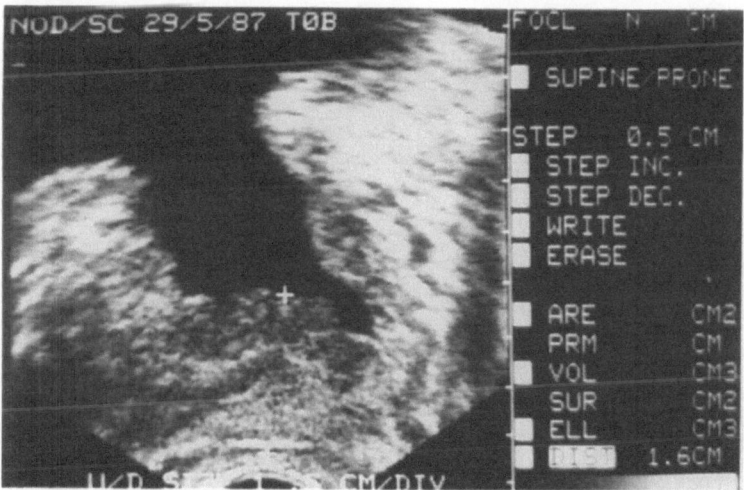

Fig. 4.1. Sagittal transrectal scan of prostate showing resection cavity. This view is particularly useful for assessing apical tissue. (By courtesy of Mr. S. Carter.)

anterior at intervals that can be set from 0.5 cm upwards. The computerised calculating facility of the machine can be used to work out the total surface area of the prostate and the volume of the gland. The images are very informative about lesions within the main body of the gland but rather less informative about the apical tissue than is the recently introduced sagittal scanning probe (Bruel and Kjaer) which gives a longitudinal cut through the prostate from apex to base of the prostate, seminal vesicles and bladder. The sagittal scan is particularly informative about the apical tissue, its extent and the characteristic extension of the peripheral zone described by McNeal (1969) at the level of the verumontanum and frequently extending below the level of the verumontanum (Fig. 4.1). Additionally, the site of the pelvic floor musculature can be readily identified.

Each patient then underwent examination under anaesthesia (EUA) followed by a second-look or "extended" TURP carefully done in planned and mapped segments. The purpose of this was firstly to "debulk" the prostate gland under ultrasound control aiming to leave a residual rim of prostatic capsule 6 mm or less in depth (Fig. 4.2.). The procedure also allows further pathological staging. Practical points will now be covered in detail.

The prostate is resected in quadrants. In addition apical specimens are taken, thus giving five segments in all. All chips are examined and the number of chips involved, the weight resected, and the Gleason scoring both per segment and overall are recorded. Using the criteria previously applied in this unit (Ford et al. 1984) those with 5% or less of the resected tissue involved by adenocarcinoma were defined as having focal or T_{0a} disease whereas those with greater than 5% involvement had diffuse or T_{0b} disease.

Finally, when the cystoscope or resectoscope is in position, the anatomical features can be defined on the ultrasound image with great confidence by placing the resectoscope loop or "rolly ball" on the peak of the verumontanum and then at the level of the endoscopically visible distal sphincter. By these means,

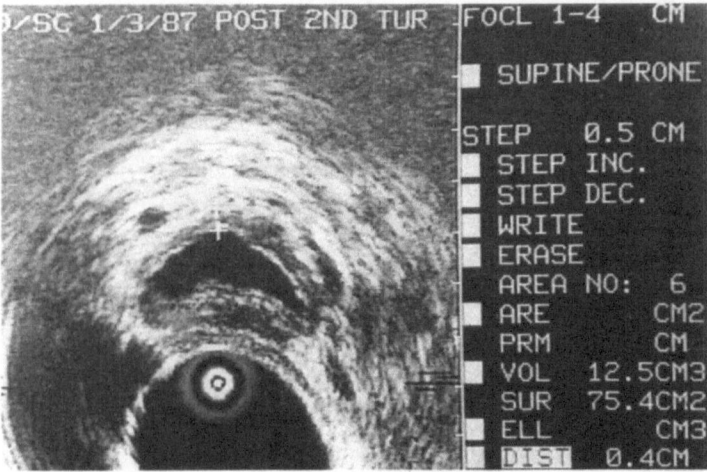

Fig. 4.2. Axial transrectal ultrasound scan showing suitable thickness of residual tissue. (By courtesy of Mr. C. Charig.)

and by the use of the measuring facilities of the ultrasound machine, very accurate measurements can be made of the amount of tissue remaining, the depth of tissue between the resected surface and the outer limit of the true capsule, and, more crucially, between the limit of resection apically and the proximal margin of the sphincter mechanism. Ultrasound assessment also allows the biopsy of suspicious areas under ultrasound control.

Ten weeks after the extended TURP the patients undergo laser coagulation of the prostatic capsule using the YAG laser. The energy is conducted along a fine quartz glass fibre that is passed down the cystoscope or resectoscope and the whole surface of the capsular walls is irradiated using a power of 50 W or, when experience increased, 60–70 W, slowly moving over the surface of the prostatic capsule in an attempt to coagulate the whole area evenly. The laser beam rests on any particular site for no more than 3–4 seconds at a time, giving a depth of penetration of the laser energy of approximately 6 mm (Pensel et al. 1981). Rectal temperatures are monitored by means of a thermocouple held against the anterior wall of the rectum behind the prostate. If the temperature reaches 52 °C the laser is stopped and the flow of irrigant increased. In practice the "educated finger" in the rectum will indicate almost as accurately when laser action should stop: it becomes too uncomfortable to maintain in position due to the temperature reached! (C. Charig 1988, personal communication.)

Transurethral access allows adequate exposure of much of the prostatic capsule and of the bladder neck. However, for good access to the apical regions a suprapubic approach is necessary. We have adapted the well-known technique of percutaneous access to the kidney to allow the creation of a dilated track into the bladder. This is followed by the passage of a specially designed access cannula through which a range of endoscopes can be passed into the bladder and into the resected prostatic cavity, allowing excellent access to the apical regions of the prostate (McNicholas et al. 1988b):

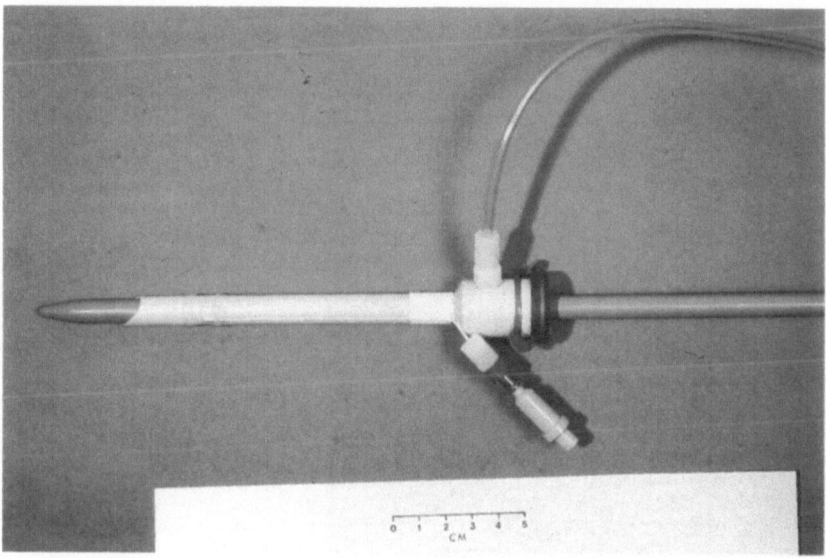

Fig. 4.3. St. Peter's Hospital cannula (Cook Urological).

1. The patient is prepared and draped for cystoscopy as usual. A small area of the lower abdomen is exposed and prepared as for suprapubic open surgery or retropubic prostatectomy. A 1-cm skin incision is made in the midline suprapubically.

2. A 12FG intravenous (i.v.) cannula and needle are inserted through the incision after palpation of the (full) bladder. If the bladder is not full or otherwise easily palpable then its position can be determined by using fluoroscopy and a small amount of contrast medium injected through a fine needle. Generally a puncture high on the anterior wall of the bladder makes access to the apical prostate and urethra easier.

3. Once urine is seen escaping from the i.v. cannula a "floppy" tipped guide wire is inserted well into the bladder.

4. The i.v. cannula is removed and a series of Teflon fascial dilators or, more commonly in our series, a set of telescopic metal dilators are passed over the guide wire to dilate a track up to 28–32Fr in calibre.

Whilst simple Amplatz-type access cannulae were used initially, these resulted in excessive soaking of the patient due to irrigant escaping from the open end of the cannula. In addition there was a risk of the cannula slipping out of the bladder. Therefore the "St. Peter's Hospital cannula" (Cook Urological, USA: Fig. 4.3) was designed to reduce still further the possibility of extravasation and to prevent inadvertent withdrawal from the bladder. It also allows controlled escape of irrigant through drainage tubing attached to a port on the proximal end, so maintaining a low-pressure irrigating system and keeping the patient dry. Its wide internal diameter (28–30Fr) allows the whole range of urological endoscopes, both rigid and flexible, to be passed as required without any risk of urethral injury either from the passage of large instruments or as a result of their repeated insertion and removal.

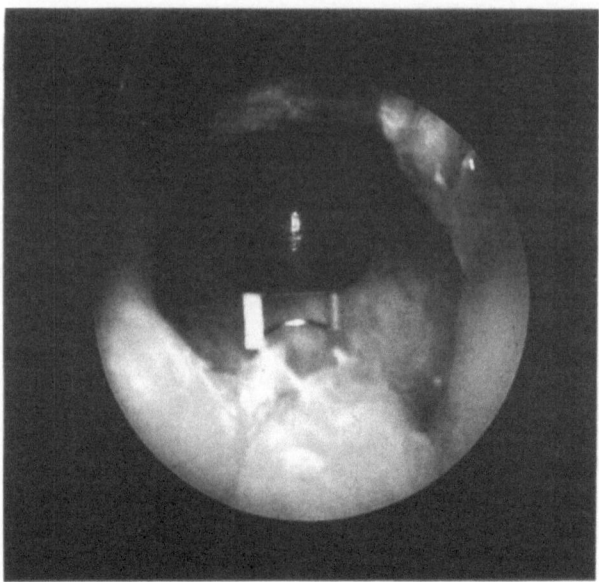

Fig. 4.4. Endoscopic view from the urethra of the suprapubic laser resectoscope.

5. Finally the St. Peter's cannula is passed over the largest dilator and enters the bladder. Gentle rotation with downward pressure is enough to push the dilators (and subsequently the cannula) into the bladder. Care is taken not to push instruments too firmly against the back wall of the bladder. The guide wire can now be removed or left as a "safety wire".

6. The balloon on the St. Peter's cannula is blown up and the cannula pulled back so that the balloon abuts the bladder wall. This reduces still further any possible extravasation and guards against inadvertently pulling the cannula from the bladder and losing the track.

7. Endoscopy with the appropriate instrument(s) and laser coagulation of the distal apical prostatic tissue can then take place (Fig. 4.4).

8. At the completion of the procedure a catheter is passed transurethrally. Its position can be checked suprapubically and then a suprapubic catheter can be placed if necessary or the cannula is removed and one silk suture used to close the skin.

9. The urethral catheter is left in the patient's bladder for a minimum of 36 hours and the patient goes home usually on the fourth day.

Post-treatment Assessment

After laser treatment patients were assessed at 1 month to confirm that they were progressing satisfactorily and were admitted for a full clinical, ultrasonic and endoscopic assessment at 3 months, 6 months and 1 year following treatment. Any problems with urinary flow or control were investigated. Potency was assessed and serological tests for serum acid phosphatase, prostate specific antigen and alkaline phosphatase were performed. Patients underwent EUA and endoscopy to monitor the healing of the prostatic capsule, in particular the bladder neck.

Ultrasound-guided biopsies of any abnormal area and "blind" transrectal prostatic biopsies of each lobe were taken in a determined effort to detect any cancer present.

The accuracy of biopsy is improved by the use of spring-loaded biopsy guns such as the "Biopty", which allows the operator to concentrate on accurate placement of the needle tip, either by digital assessment of the suspicious area or by using ultrasound guidance, after which the safety catch can be released and the biopsy taken. This avoids the inaccuracies due to the relatively coarse movements resulting from manipulation of a "Tru-cut" biopsy needle.

Blind biopsies are taken transrectally, the patient being given prophylactic antibiotic cover with gentamicin intravenously and metronidazole rectally. Ultrasound-guided biopsies are performed transperineally as the ultrasound axial transducer occupies the rectum and the computerised needle "guide-lines" projected onto the ultrasound image on the screen assume a transperineal approach. (The newer sagittal scanning probes allow transrectal biopsy.) Any suspicious area was biopsied and in the absence of clinical or ultrasound suspicion a representative biopsy was taken of each lobe of the posterior prostate. Subsequently patients were seen in the prostate clinic and underwent an annual bone scan.

Results

Twenty-five males have undergone a complete course of treatment (extended TURP followed by laser coagulation of the prostatic cavity) since April 1986. As a result of the staging procedures a further four have been excluded: one because of lymph node involvement found at pelvioscopy, two relatively unfit males with T_{0a} disease confirmed on second-look TURP and one because of severe coexisting illness.

The average of all patients was 63.5 years (range 39–76) and of the laser patients 62.4 years (range 39–75). Results of the pathological assessment of the tissue removed when a first TURP was performed compared with that removed at the subsequent extended TURP is shown in Table 4.1. Table 4.2 shows similar

Table 4.1. Comparison of pathological assessment of prostatic tissue removed in patients undergoing both first TURP and "extended" TURP ($n = 13$)

	Positive histology	Gleason score (Mean and range)	Focal or no disease[a] (No. and %)	Diffuse disease[b] (No. and %)	% chips positive (Mean and range)	Weight resected (g) (Mean and range)
First TURP	13	2.9 (2–6)	6 (46%)	7 (54%)	9.2% (1–25)	21 (4–56)
"Extended" TURP	11	3.5 (0–6)	6 (46%)	7 (54%)	8% (0–25)	12.3 (1.5–21)

[a]5% or less of chips positive (Ford et al. 1984).
[b]More than 5% of chips positive.

Table 4.2. Pathological assessment of prostatic tissue removed by "extended" TURP ($n = 20$)

Positive histology	Gleason score (Mean and range)	Focal or no disease[a] (No. and %)	Diffuse disease[b] (No. and %)	% chips positive (Mean and range)	Weight resected (g) (Mean and range)
16	4 (2–7)	7 (35%)	13 (65%)	11% (0–75)	13.2 (1.5–26)

[a]5% or less of chips positive (Ford et al. 1984).
[b]More than 5% of chips positive.

Table 4.3. Clinical. pathological and ultrasound staging ($n = 20$)

	T_0		T_1	T_2	T_3
	T_{0a}	T_{0b}			
Clinical		11	6	3	0
Pathological	4	7			
Ultrasound		6	9	3	2

details of the pathological findings from 20 males undergoing extended TURP. Disease stage of the 20 patients is detailed according to their clinical, pathological and ultrasonic features in Table 4.3 and energy doses administered per treatment are illustrated in Fig. 4.5.

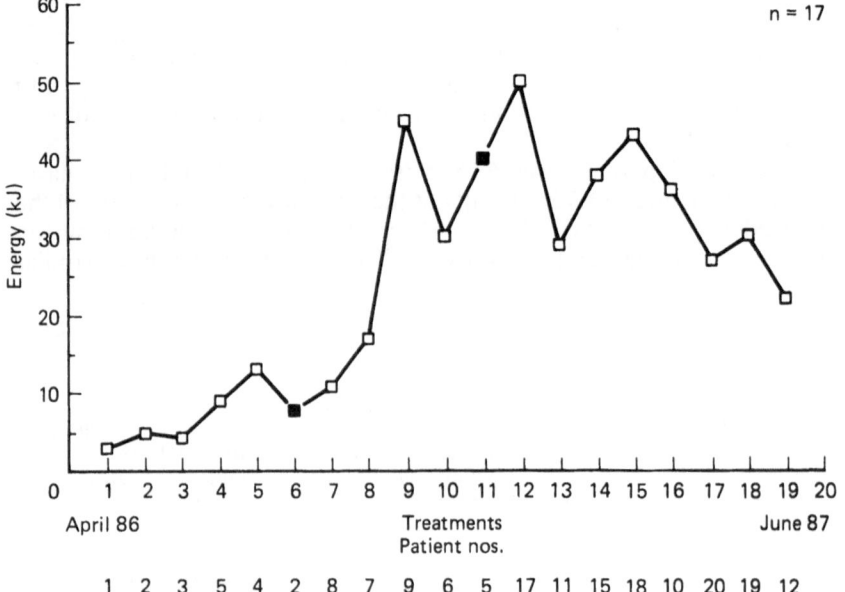

Fig. 4.5. Graph showing energy given per treatment during the early development of the technique. Filled squares indicate second treatments.

In the immediate post-TURP period one patient complained of urgency, two described perineal discomfort and one required a 2-unit blood transfusion after his extended TURP. No other patient required transfusion and the average inpatient stay was 4 days. One patient subsequently described the passage of clots with no other sequelae whilst at home awaiting his laser treatment. Another patient described a diminution of flow after his extended TURP and at laser treatment was noted to have a degree of bladder neck obstruction. This same patient was seen to have a much more marked degree of bladder neck obstruction 3 months after his laser treatment and underwent bladder neck incision with subsequent relief of his symptoms and improvement in his flow rate.

After laser treatment four patients described perineal discomfort in the first 3 months. (The perineal discomfort previously reported by one patient prior to laser treatment did not recur after the treatment.) These patients had all received much higher energy doses than previously used as we gradually increased the total energy dose as experience increased (see Fig. 4.5). At their 3-month follow-up three patients had a large amount of slough in the prostatic cavity; this was removed with the resectoscope loop to avoid any possible dystrophic calcification. This tissue was avascular and did not bleed. Four patients were noted to have a mild bladder neck stenosis not requiring treatment and two had a more marked but asymptomatic bladder neck stenosis. They both underwent bladder neck incision at their 3-month endoscopy and one of them required a repeat bladder neck incision on one occasion subsequently.

There were no immediate alterations to continence or potency with the exception of one patient who has had no erections since laser treatment and had not been sexually active prior to treatment. He had described a reduction in erections after his extended TURP. One other patient complained of reduced quality of erections after treatment, but the clinical features of early prostate cancer had been a chance finding during investigation of this problem and other studies suggested a psychogenic cause for his erectile dysfunction. Follow-up now extends to over 3 years for the early members of the group and within the last 3 months one 59-year-old man has been reviewed and complains of deteriorating erections. He is currently being investigated further.

In the early stages of follow-up two patients had positive biopsies. In both cases clinical, ultrasonic and endoscopic evidence suggested that an excess of tissue had been left. They have both undergone further debulking TURP and second laser treatments with negative biopsies subsequently. Two patients have clinical and pathological evidence of remaining apical disease: in retrospect they were understaged despite our best efforts and would not have been suitable for any local therapy given with curative intent. The other patients have negative biopsies. In no case has disease progressed.

After extended TURP, ultrasound images characteristically showed a thin hyperechoic area on the resected surface and this characteristic picture was repeated and exaggerated after the laser treatment. This does have the disadvantage that ultrasound assessment of these patients is particularly difficult after the extended TURP (and, of course, they may also have undergone a primary diagnostic TURP) especially when followed by laser treatment. Characteristically the whole gland is much shrunken, both in total length and in its anteroposterior diameter (Fig. 4.6).

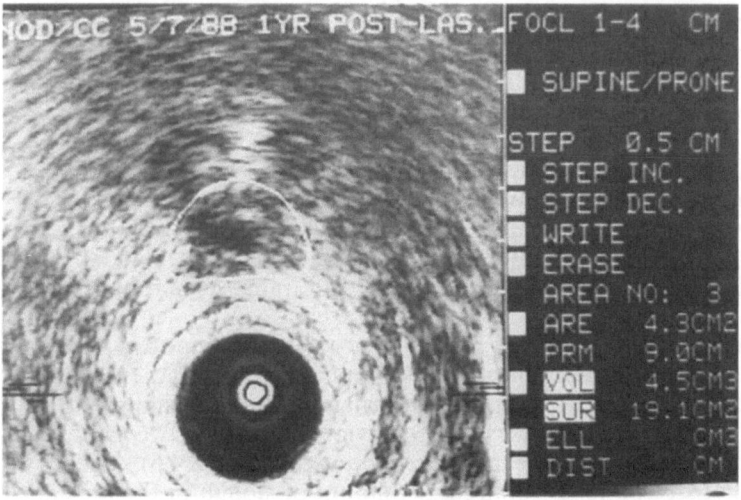

Fig. 4.6. Transrectal ultrasound scan showing foreshortened prostate after laser treatment and radical TURP (volume 4.5 ml). (By courtesy of Mr. C. Charig.)

Discussion and Conclusions

Radical Endoscopic Local Treatment

There have been previous attempts at either endoscopic treatment of carcinoma of the prostate or other surgical methods short of complete radical retropubic or perineal prostatectomy. One such was reported by Riches in 1970, who described his methods of removing the posterior lobe of the prostate including capsule at open retropubic surgery as a prophylactic measure when there was a suspicion of prostatic cancer. This method does not address the fact that tumour may well exist in anterior and lateral parts of the prostate (Eggleston and Walsh 1985).

An endoscopic "extensive" or "radical" TURP with the intention of removing all prostatic tissue, both adenoma and true prostatic gland tissue, leaving only the prostatic capsule, is fraught with technical problems. Most importantly there are the difficulties in truly removing all the tissue that is intended for removal; secondly, severe haemorrhage from pericapsular vessels may be encountered. The method described here overcomes these problems by allowing an extensive ultrasound-guided resection that remains generally within the bounds of the prostate but allows complete coagulation of the residual prostatic "rim" by means of the laser. Tissues beyond the prostate, including the pelvic autonomic nerves, may be protected by the "heat sink" effect of the pericapsular and more distant vessels; diathermy, in contrast, may be relatively concentrated on these vascular channels, leading to the potential for concentration of current and resultant thermal injury. In laser treatment the rectum is also protected by the presence of Denonvilliers' fascia (and the pelvic plexus nerves responsible for potency may be protected by the vasa nervorum and the veins of Santorini's plexus).

Effects on Prostate

The prostatic shrinkage that characterises this treatment has not been reported by the other group with any experience in this field, though they do report the characteristic increase in hyperechoic lesions within the prostate (Beisland and Laerum 1986). It is clear from discussions with Dr. Beisland and from their reported works (Sander and Beisland 1984) that the energy levels they use are distinctly lower than ours, which may account for this difference in the final appearances of the gland.

Whatever the ultrasound appearance of the abnormal area, final confirmation of the presence of tumour is by biopsy and pathological assessment of the material. Dr. Beisland's group does not routinely biopsy patients post-operatively if the clinical and ultrasound appearances do not suggest malignancy. We have found this potentially misleading, and biopsy all patients post-operatively as described above. Dr. Beisland describes a small decrease in the maximal transverse diameter of the capsule in the first 3–6 months after laser treatment with little additional shrinkage from that time (Beisland and Laerum 1986). Our experience has been the opposite, and many of our patients have a marked shrinkage of the prostate both in the anteroposterior diameter and in the length of the gland – so much so that endoscopically the trigone seems to be approaching the verumontanum! It is not clear, though, whether this is due to the combination of (frequently) two resections, or largely a result of the laser treatment. Our patients frequently showed a marked hyperechoic area on the surface of the prostatic urethra. This was particularly the case in those who had a marked degree of necrotic slough on the luminal surface at the 3-month endoscopy; it was also noted to a lesser degree in some patients after TURP.

Ultrasonic Assessment of Treatment

One of the problems encountered during the study was how best to follow up the patients with a view to recognising recurrence. The volume of the gland after laser treatment is so small as to render it almost impalpable, and blind biopsy usually fails to show any evidence of prostatic tissue, the biopsy needle tending to pass into the seminal vesicles. We have now become familiar with the characteristic transrectal ultrasound appearances of the gland after treatment. The gland is very small and rounded, with a very echodense capsule and periurethral area; there is loss of the normal architecture and an extremely foreshortened prostatic urethra. The sagittal viewing ultrasound probe has been very useful in performing post-treatment ultrasounds. We have found the axial scanner can only take one or at most two slices through the gland due to the extremely shortened prostatic length. With recognition of the patterns described and accurate biopsy, it is possible to be fairly certain that residual tumour is not being missed.

At the time of endoscopic assessment blind prostatic biopsies of each lobe are taken by a transrectal biopsy. Biopsies are also taken under ultrasound control. This can mean that patients have up to six biopsies in an attempt to get an accurate histopathological assessment of their prostatic glands and the presence of tumour. These extensive attempts to determine the presence or absence of tumour have not resulted in any clinically noticeable morbidity. In contrast to other studies (Beisland and Laerum 1986) positive biopsies are taken as a sign of failure of the treatment rather than, by analogy with the argument used in some radiotherapeutic studies (Cox and Stoffel 1977), a sign that the process of tumour necrosis as a result of the therapeutic insult may be a lengthy one, especially in a relatively slow-growing tumour.

This series has allowed us to watch the volume changes during the stages of the treatment and during follow-up. The average volume of the gland at diagnosis was 24.4 ml (range 17–38 ml) and after the second-look or extended TURP, 14 ml (range 9.4–22.3 ml); at 3 months after laser treatment the mean volume of the glands was 7.5 ml (range 2.3–19.5 ml). Overall, therefore, there is a 71% reduction in volume of the prostate gland.

Prostate Specific Antigen

The recent introduction of the prostate specific antigen (PSA) assay is a possible major advance in the determination of the extent of prostatic cancer, and in the monitoring of the response of prostatic cancer to treatment.

We have performed PSA studies following laser treatment in a total of 23 patients. In 14, values measured at least 6 months after treatment have dropped into the same range as that following successful total prostatectomy for localised disease (<0.5 µg/l). In two patients the level is 0.5 µg/l, in three between 0.5 and 2 µg/l, and in one between 2 and 4 µg/l. Levels in a further three patients are above 4 µg/l, including the two patients previously mentioned who had extensive local disease at the time of endoscopic laser treatment.

Second-look TURP and the Dissemination of Disease

The possibility that TURP and in particular a second-look, radical or extended TURP such as described above could have an adverse influence on the prognosis of prostatic cancer, has to be considered. It is conceivable that particularly as the outer limits of the prostate are reached, and the effects of treatment tend to impinge on the relatively large-bore, low-pressure venous sinuses, then viable tumour cell material could be liberated and might find its way into these vessels and thence disseminate. Dissemination of viable prostatic tumour cells after TURP has been reported by Cole et al. (1961), who found cancer cells in the inferior vena cava following TURP; similarly Miedena and Redman (1981) found pulmonary emboli of prostatic cancer, believed to be a direct result of TURP.

In 1980 McGowan noted an increased recurrence rate in patients treated with radiation therapy for early stages B and C (American staging system) prostatic cancers when diagnosis had been by transurethral resection rather than needle biopsy. Hanks et al. (1983) were able to review 690 patients with cancer of the prostate, staged according to the American Joint Committee system, who had undergone radiation therapy in 1973 with curative intent. Of these, 247 cases were excluded from the analysis either because of incomplete data or because they were T_0 or had evidence of existing disease prior to treatment. The remaining 443 were evaluated to assess whether TURP had an adverse effect on the progress of those cases where the diagnosis was made by TURP rather than needle biopsy.

A statistical analysis was performed in which the expected frequency of local recurrence, recurrence anywhere and death, were calculated for each stage of prostatic cancer and then compared with the observed frequencies. The figures revealed an adverse effect of TURP in patients with T_3 and T_4 cancers (the two stages being combined together in the actuarial analysis). The local recurrence rate was unaffected, but the rate of recurrence anywhere and the death rate were increased. These effects were seen for moderately and poorly differentiated tumours, but were not observed in any well-differentiated cancers of any stage. In addition, there was a clear increase in the number of poorly differentiated cancers in the TURP group compared with the needle biopsy group, and a corresponding increase in well-differentiated cancers in the needle biopsy group compared with the TURP group.

Against this finding can be put the probability that tumours continuously embolise cells via lymphatics and blood regardless of whether external manipulation is present. It remains to be shown whether the presence of circulating tumour cells *per se* is a poor prognostic feature. Metastasis is the end point of a complex sequence of events that involves host and tumour factors. Studies have failed to show that normal shedding of cells into the blood stream during manipulation results in metastatic disease. However, it may well be that like is not being compared with like. It is quite possible that, since fairly advanced tumours in the studies by Hanks et al. seem to show this deleterious effect of TURP, these patients have a larger volume of tumour in their prostates. This means tumour is more likely to be present in a transurethral resection specimen, and of course is also more likely to be present already in lymph nodes and more distant sites.

Schwemmer et al. (1986), in a study of 122 patients with prostatic carcinoma treated by radiation therapy, performed a similar actuarial analysis on survival, comparing those treated by transurethral resection prior to radiation with those diagnosed by needle biopsy. Survival rates were not significantly different between the groups, and TURP was not found to have any effect on the disease-free interval, whether distant or local recurrence occurred. From a multivariate analysis model that allowed adjustments for the effects of tumour grade and stage, TURP was found to be without effect on either survival rates or the interval to distant or local recurrence.

Levine et al. (1986) reviewed 415 patients with prostatic carcinoma treated between 1965 and 1971, of whom 184 were evaluable. They were assessed for the impact of TURP at each stage. There was no significant difference between a TURP diagnosed group and a group diagnosed by needle biopsy in stage A, C or D, though in stage B the 5-year survival difference between the TURP group (38.7%) and the needle biopsy group (68%) was significant. These authors do comment that clinical staging may be inaccurate, and that the stage of the lymph nodes was unknown. They referred to the study by Fowler et al. (1982) in which 58 patients subsequently receiving iodine-125 implantations had undergone TURP within the previous 10 months.

Fowler et al.'s most striking finding was that the incidence of positive lymph node metastasis was greater in the patients who had undergone TURP than in those who had not (47% compared with 25%). Survival without distant metastases for stage B tumours appeared to be greater amongst those patients without prior TURP, suggesting that the procedure may have been harmful. However, patients with stage C tumours who had undergone TURP appeared to have a higher probability of survival without metastasis. The data suggested that patients with localised carcinoma of the prostate (B) were more likely to have lymph node metastases already.

It is quite possible that the patients who were diagnosed by TURP had larger tumours perhaps causing the obstructive symptoms, which tended to suggest to the surgeon the need for TURP as a means of diagnosis as well as therapy rather than just needle biopsy. From this review it is to be concluded that there is little identifiable risk from the procedure as described by our group and by Sander and Beisland.

It is too early to make any suggestion as to the overall efficacy of this technique. In addition, the method has been altered in the light of our increasing experience. Fig. 4.5 shows the steady increase in total energy given as confidence in the technique increased, and as we became aware that the earliest patients had been relatively undertreated. These energy totals are much higher than those described by Beisland et al. (personal communication 1988), but we consider them essential to the reliable achievement of a sufficiently deep effect over the whole surface area of the prostatic cavity. The extent of resection increased in a similar fashion, both with increasing familiarity with the ultrasound guidance and in the light of subsequent evidence that, again, the earliest patients had been inadequately resected. 17 patients underwent a complete course of treatment in the pilot study (1985–87).

The combination of inadequate resection and inadequate laser treatment resulted in the two early treatment failures. (These have since been successfully re-treated, with negative serial biopsies.) However, the method in its present state of development has resulted in 88% (15 of 17) of the treated patients having no evidence of disease despite careful and repeated biopsy and EUA. The two remaining treatment failures (11.8%) had residual tumour in the apical region of the gland. Apical tissue remains a challenge to this method of treatment. It is known to be often the site of tumour (Byar and Mostofi 1972) and this part of the prostate may be difficult to resect completely by the transurethral route without compromising the external sphincter. Our attention is currently being directed to more radical methods of performing the final resection of apical tissue, both from below and from the suprapubic track. All resection is guided by the ultrasound image, on which the sphincter and resectoscope can both be clearly identified.

Although any treatment for carcinoma of the prostate must be judged over a prolonged period of follow-up, the treatment described can be repeated, has not affected continence and results, in our experience, in a low incidence of impotence.

Carcinoma of the Penis

Penile cancer remains a relatively unusual disease in the Western world. Standard treatment remains penile amputation or radiotherapy. The extent of the amputation is dependent on the local extent of the tumour. Obviously this procedure is mutilating and will have effects on the patient's psyche and also on his voiding. Radiotherapy is suitable for localised lesions and as a palliative option. It may be quite painful and may result in urethral stenosis. For superficial tumours of the penis laser methods may be as effective as the standard treatments and less mutilating.

The YAG laser would appear to be the most appropriate laser for treating certain penile carcinomas because of its greater depth of penetration. Hofstetter and Frank (1983) have reported their experience of its use to treat 17 patients with penile cancer who had refused standard surgical therapy. Re-epithelialisation took place in 6–8 weeks and the authors described excellent cosmetic results. Eleven of the patients were followed for at least 10 months and only one suffered local recurrence. Malloy et al. (1988) treated 16 males with squamous cell cancer of the penis who had refused amputation. They irradiated the tumours with a YAG laser at 25–40 W, giving an average of 5000 J. At follow-up 24 months later those with carcinoma *in situ* did very well, with no evidence of recurrent tumour. The details of the T_1 patients are somewhat unclear though most were disease free (6 of 9); however both T_2 patients had residual disease despite the deeper penetration of the YAG laser.

However, Bandeiramonte et al. (1987, 1988) have more recently described a method of microscopic surgery with the CO_2 laser for the excision of superficial penile cancers. They used magnification to allow accurate assessment of the extent and depth of the tumour in 15 patients and then treated the pathological area by firing a CO_2 laser (at 20 W) through the microscope to vaporise layers of the abnormal tissue until healthy tissue was reached.

It would appear that either the CO_2 or YAG laser is suitable for treating superficial malignant lesions of the penis and indeed for usually superficial but preneoplastic conditions such as erythroplasia of Queyrat and Bowen's disease (Rosemberg and Fuller 1980). The choice may therefore be guided by the instruments available. Laser treatment of more invasive disease must be regarded as an experimental procedure at present.

Our patients have been treated similarly to those described by Hofstetter and Frank (1983). Their patients were first circumcised and a tourniquet placed around the base of the penis to decrease bleeding during treatment. After excision of exophytic tumour, the tumour bed and a 0.5-cm margin around it were treated with 2-second laser pulses at 40 W. We take care to coagulate whilst cooling the penile surface with a stream of cold saline. This increases the depth of effect by preventing charring on the surface (which would increase the surface absorption of energy and reduce the deeper penetration and subsequent scattering of laser light). The tourniquet is then released to allow full haemostasis.

It has proved essential to excise the protuberant tumour tissue. Presumably this allows an adequate depth of tumour necrosis. At the same time the operative site has to be kept free of blood, which would also reduce the depth of effective necrosis. Biopsy or excision of exophytic tissue has therefore to be performed after the application of the tourniquet. Diathermy or suture haemostasis may be necessary in addition.

It is important to delineate the extent of tumour as accurately and completely as possible so as to ensure that all malignant tissue is coagulated. This may not be easy, especially when the penis has received previous radiation treatment. This problem did lead to treatment "failure" in one of our patients. His obvious tumour recurrence on the glans penis was adequately coagulated using the YAG laser (Fig. 4.7) with a good cosmetic result at 3 months, but soon

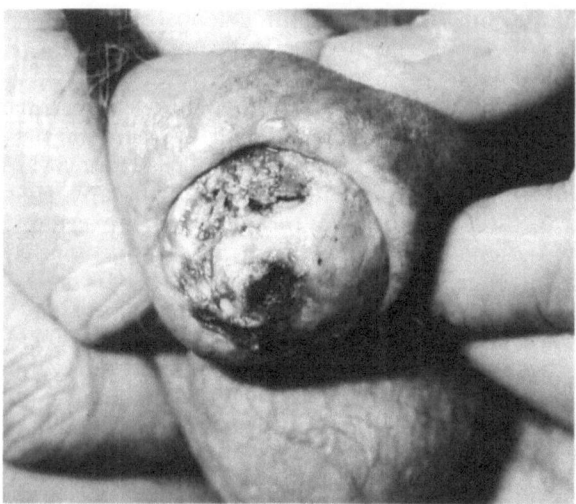

Fig. 4.7. Appearances after YAG laser coagulation of recurrent penile cancer following radiotherapy.

after he developed further recurrent tumour on the foreskin at the peno-
glanular junction in an area that had not received laser treatment (Fig. 4.8).

Laser treatment may avoid the need for partial penectomy in those patients
with recurrence after radiotherapy. In our experience patients report that the
treatment is generally more comfortable than external beam radiotherapy. The
main problem we have found is that it takes some weeks for the necrotic laser
eschar to separate and care is necessary to avoid infection and to ensure a dry
eschar.

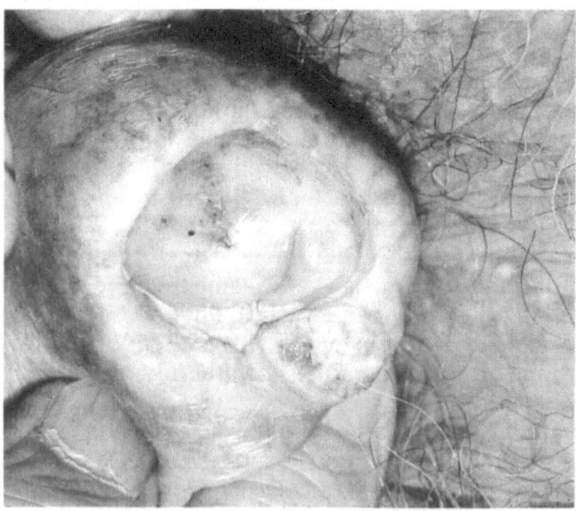

Fig. 4.8. Recurrent tumour on foreskin outside laser-treated area. Treated glans has healed well.
(By courtesy of Mr. C.A. Charlton.)

References

Prostate

Adami H-O, Norlen BJ, Malker B, Meirik O (1986) Long term survival in prostatic carcinoma with special reference to age as a prognostic factor. Scand J Urol Nephrol 20:107–112

Beisland HO, Laerum F (1986) Transrectal ultrasonography before and after neodymium YAG laser irradiation of localised prostatic carcinoma. Eur Urol 12 [Suppl 1]:39–42

Beisland HO, Sander S (1986) First clinical experiences on neodymium-YAG laser irradiation of localised prostatic carcinoma. Scand J Urol Nephrol 20:113–117

Beynon LL, Busuttil A, Newsam JE, Chisholm GD (1983) Incidental carcinoma of the prostate: selection for deferred treatment. Br J Urol 55:733–736

Byar DP, Mostofi FK (1972) Carcinoma of the prostate: prognostic evaluation of certain pathologic features in 208 radical prostatectomies. Cancer 30:5–13

Cantrell BB, De Klerk DP, Eggleston JC, Boitnott JK, Walsh PC (1981) Pathological factors that influence prognosis in stage A prostatic cancer: the influence of extent versus grade. J Urol 125:516–520

Carter SSt, Peeling B, Fellows G, Whipp E, O'Donoghue EPN (1987) Ultrasound guided transperineal ^{125}I seed implantation for prostatic cancer. Paper read at British Association of Urological Surgeons meeting, Edinburgh, July 1987

Chisholm GD, Habib FK (1981) Prostatic cancer: experimental and clinical advances. In: Hendry WF (ed) Recent advances in urology/andrology 3. Churchill Livingstone, Edinburgh, pp 211–232

Cole WH, McDonald GO, Roberts SS, Southwick HW (1961) Dissemination of cancer: prevention and therapy. Appleton-Century-Crofts, New York, p 143

Cox JD, Stoffel TJ (1977) The significance of needle biopsy after irradiation for stage C adenocarcinoma of the prostate. Cancer 40:156–160

Eggleston JC, Walsh, PC (1985) Radical prostatectomy with preservation of sexual function: pathological findings in the first 100 cases. J Urol 134:1146–1148

Ford TF, Cameron KM, Parkinson CM, O'Donoghue EPN (1984) Incidental carcinoma of the prostate: treatment selection by second-look TURP. Br J Urol 56:682–686

Fordham MVP, Burdget AH, Matthews J, Williams G, Cooke T (1986) Prostatic carcinoma cell DNA content measured by flow cytometry and its relation to clinical outcome. Br J Surg 73:400–403

Fowler JE, Fisher HAG, Kiser DL, Whitmore WF (1982) Pelvic lymph node metastases and probability of survival without distant metastases in patients treated with ^{125}I implantation for localised prostatic cancer: influence of pretreatment transurethral resection of the prostate. Paper presented at the 77th Annual Meeting of the American Urological Association, Kansas City, 16–20 May

Franks LM (1954) Latent carcinoma of the prostate. J Pathol Bacteriol 68:603–616

Gleason DF, Mellinger GT and the Veterans Administration Cooperative Urological Research Group (1974) Prediction of prognosis for prostatic adenocarcinoma by combined histological grading and clinical staging. J Urol 111:58–64

Goldstein I, Feldman M, Deckers PJ, Babayan RK, Krane RJ (1984) Radiation associated impotence: a clinical study of its mechanism. JAMA 251:903–910

Hanks GE, Leibel S, Kramer S (1983) Dissemination of cancer by transurethral resection of locally advanced prostate cancer. J Urol 129:309–311

Harty JI, Blicblum S, Amin M (1979) In vitro technique for isolating prostatic cells from blood. J Surg Res 26:411–416

Jewett HJ (1975) The present status of radical prostatectomy for stages A and B prostatic cancer. Urol Clin N Am 2:105–124

Levine ES, Sisek VJ, Mulvihill MN, Cohen EL (1986) The role of transurethral resection in dissemination of cancer of the prostate. Urology 28:179–183

Lindholt J, Hansen TP (1986) Prostatic carcinoma: complications of megavoltage radiation therapy. Br J Urol 58:52–54

McGowan DG (1980) The adverse influence of prior TUR in prognosis of carcinoma of the prostate treated by radiotherapy. Int J Radiat Oncol Biol Phys 6:1121–1124

McNeal JE (1969) Origin and development of carcinoma in the prostate. Cancer 23:24–34

McNeal JE, Kindrachuk RA, Freiha FS, Bostwick DG, Redwine EA, Stamey TA (1986) Patterns of progression in prostate cancer. Lancet i:60–63

McNicholas TA, Carter SStC, Wickham JEA, O'Donoghue EPN (1988a) YAG laser treatment of early carcinoma of the prostate. Br J Urol 61:239–243

McNicholas TA, Ramsay JWA, Carter SStC, Miller RA (1988b) Suprapubic endoscopy: a percutaneous approach. Br J Urol 61:221–223

Miedena EB, Redman JF (1981) Microscopic pulmonary embolisation by adenocarcinoma of the prostate. Urology 18:399

Mostofi FK (1975) Grading of prostatic cancer. Cancer Chemother Rep 59:111

Nag S (1985) Radioactive I-125 implantation for carcinoma of the prostate. The Prostate 6:293–301

Newman AJ, Graham MA, Carlton CE, Lieman S (1982) Incidental carcinoma of the prostate at the time of transurethral resection: importance of evaluating every chip. J Urol 128:948–950

Parkin DM, Stjernsward J, Muir CS (1984) Estimates of the worldwide frequency of twelve major cancers. Bull WHO 62:163–182

Paulson DF (1980) Assessment of anatomic extent and biologic hazard of prostatic adenocarcinoma. Urology 25:537–541

Pensel J, Hofstetter A, Keiditsch E, Rothenberger K (1981) Temporal and spatial temperature profile of the bladder serosa in intravesical neodymium YAG laser irradiation. Eur Urol 7:298–303

Ray GR, Bagshaw MA (1975) The role of radiation therapy in the definitive treatment of adenocarcinoma of the prostate. Annu Rev Med 26:567–588

Riches EW (1970) Prophylaxis of carcinoma of the prostate. Mod Trends Urol 3:264–278

Ritchie AWS, Smith G, Preston C, Beynon LL, Duncan W, Chisholm GD (1985) Prediction of response to radiotherapy for localised prostatic cancer. Br J Urol 57:729–732

Sander S, Beisland HO (1984) Laser in the treatment of localised prostatic carcinoma. J Urol 132:280–281

Sander S, Beisland HO, Fossberg E (1982) Neodymium YAG laser in the treatment of prostatic cancer. Urol Res 10:85–86

Schwemmer B, Ulm K, Rotter M, Braen J, Schutz W (1986) Does transurethral resection of prostatic carcinoma promote tumour spread? Urol Int 41:284–288

Sheldon CA, Williams RD, Fraley EE (1980) Incidental carcinoma of the prostate: a review of the literature and critical reappraisal of classification. J Urol 124:626–631

Smith JM, Kelly DG (1984) Radical prostatectomy in the management of localised carcinoma of the prostate. Br J Urol 56:690–693

UICC (1978) TNM classification of malignant tumours. Union International Contre le Cancer, Geneva

Walsh PC, Jewett HJ (1980) Radical surgery for prostatic cancer. Cancer 45:1906–1911

Walsh PC, Mostwin JL (1984) Radical prostatectomy and cystoprostatectomy with preservation of potency: results using a new nerve sparing technique. Br J Urol 56:694–697

Penis

Bandeiramonte G, Lepera P, Marchesini S, Andreola S, Pizzocaro G (1987) Laser microsurgery for superficial lesions of the penis. J Urol 138:315–319

Bandeiramonte G, Santoro O, Boracchi P, Piva L, Pizzocaro G, DePalo G (1988) Total resection of glans penis surface by CO_2 laser microsurgery. Acta Oncol 27:575–578

Hofstetter A, Frank F (1983) Laser use in urology. In: Dixon JA (ed) Surgical application of lasers. Year Book Publishers, Chicago, pp 146–162

Malloy TR, Wein AJ, Carpiniello VL (1988) Carcinoma of the penis treated with neodymium YAG laser. Urology 31:26–29

Rosemberg SK, Fuller T (1980) Carbon dioxide rapid superpulsed laser treatment of erythroplasia of Queyrat. Urology 16:181–182

Chapter 5

Laser Treatment of Benign Conditions of the Urinary Tract

T. A. McNicholas

Urethral Strictures

Introduction and Historical Background

The treatment of urethral strictures remains a challenge to the urologist. Whilst great advances in the instrumentation now allow endoscopic treatment for most simple strictures, there is still room for improvement and new methods of dealing with the strictured urethra will always be eagerly explored.

Urethral strictures have affected man since time immemorial. It is certainly an ancient problem and early man responded to this challenge by developing measures to relieve the obstructing stenosis by means of the passage of dilators of one sort or another. The recorded history of stricture treatment dates back to the sixth century BC, when the use of wooden or metal dilators was described in the Ayurveda. Graduated catheters of wood and metal to dilate strictures is still the most commonly used method worldwide.

Subsequently, over the last two millennia a range of methods of cutting strictures have been developed. In the sixteenth century Ambroise Paré developed a long, sharp lancet to "reduce excrescences" in the urethra. His generation felt that the stricture resulted from the ingrowth of inflammatory tissue impinging into the urethral lumen rather than a contraction of the lumen *per se*. In 1795 the appropriately named Dr Physick of Philadelphia described his lancellated catheter; this was followed in 1817 by Jean Civiale's sound with a bulb containing a blade. However, as a result of the size of the bulb only large-calibre strictures could be passed by the sound and then cut by removal of the sound with the blade now exposed. Instruments devised to perform blind urethrotomies were designed by Maisonneuve in 1854 (a filiform with urethrotome which could therefore deal with smaller-calibre strictures) and by Fessenden N. Otis in 1872. Otis developed calibrating catheters and sounds and went on to design the two-bladed dilating urethrotome with a cutting blade much as we know it today; he had high hopes that he had devised a method of curing strictures.

The direct-vision optical urethrotome was developed in the 1950s in stages, initially utilising electric diathermy (Ravasini 1957) and eventually in the form of the cold knife optical urethrotome. Sachse introduced the optical endoscopic urethrotome as it is currently known in 1974, and it is, of course, widely used as a primary treatment in most Western urological units. In the years since Sachse's publication many reports have shown the relative ease and comparative safety of this technique (Matouschek 1978; Smith et al. 1983, 1984; Djulepa and Potempa 1983; Andronaco et al. 1984).

Le Dran is reputed to have carried out the first excision of a stricture in 1744, but it is also claimed that his description could equally be that of an external urethrotomy. Ducas in 1835 can perhaps be given the credit for the first recorded excision of a urethral stricture. He relied on healing of the tissues over the underlying catheter to lead to re-formation of the urethra. Agusner carried out the first excision of the stricture with restoration of the urethral continuity by suture in 1883, closely followed by many others. Guyon in 1891 described excising part of the stricture leaving a strip of the dorsal urethral wall in continuity, and Albarran in 1892 described a similar technique. Rachet in 1895 recommended diversion of the urine during operations for stricture. Pasteau and Iselin in 1906 excised a stricture leaving the two ends of the urethra opening on to the skin. They subsequently incorporated adjacent skin into the wall of the urethra and created a skin tube.

Hamilton Russell in 1911 aimed at creating an "artificial hypospadias", excising the urethra for the whole length of the stricture, but was prevented from carrying out the "second stage" by the patient's lack of symptoms and his understandable desire to avoid further operation. In 1915 Russell excised a stricture and spatulated the ends of the remaining urethra, joining them at the ventral surface of the urethra. He explained that he relied on natural processes to reconvert the "roof" strip of mucous membrane into a tube. This is clearly the forerunner of the Denis Browne procedure for hypospadias.

In 1950 Bengt Johanson adapted the Denis Browne hypospadias operation to the treatment of adult urethral strictures, incising the strictured urethra until well into normal urethra on each side and suturing the cut edges of the urethra to the adjacent skin edges to create, in effect, an artificial hypospadias. As a second stage a strip of original urethra and adjacent penile skin was left *in situ* to form a new urethra, the rest of the skin being closed over. Variations on this theme have been multiple, including the use of pedicled scrotal skin (Blandy 1986) and pedicled penile skin patches (Turner-Warwick 1987; Mundy and Stephenson 1988). Most recently high-energy laser technology has been applied to this persisting and resistant problem.

Current Treatment Methods

Urethral dilatation is the oldest form of treatment and realistically will remain the foremost treatment for most sufferers throughout the world. It should not be lightly disregarded. In the appropriate case, whether for reasons of economy, age or the nature or position of the stricture, it will remain part of the urological armamentarium even in the richest societies where more expensive technology is available. However, a patient is rarely cured by one dilatation and is more commonly sentenced to multiple attendances and procedures, which often become more difficult and traumatic with time and carry an increasing attendant morbidity and indeed mortality.

The procedure of open urethroplasty exists as a final option and remains the "gold standard" against which other treatments, for complex strictures particularly, should be measured. However, urethroplasty is a major procedure requiring skilled technical performance, and even in the best hands there is the possibility of recurrence, especially at the junction of neourethra and urethra. In addition the patient suffers a cutaneous incision and all the complications, morbidity and discomfort of open surgery. Finally, although patients with pelvic fracture injury "strictures" are frequently impotent an additional risk of post-operative impotence in those who were previously potent has been described for transpubic urethroplasty (Zincke and Furlow 1985).

Endoscopic methods, if effective, are to be preferred, and optical urethrotomy is accepted as a good initial treatment for most simple strictures. Since the introduction of the cold knife urethrotome most simple strictures are readily treated in the first instance in this way. However, the urethrotome fails as a definitive treatment for many strictures, especially if long or complicated by sepsis, abscess and fistulae. When the underlying problem is an abundance of scar tissue the urethrotome does nothing to reduce this and may even cause an increase in periurethral fibrosis due to extravasation of (infected) urine (Singh and Blandy 1976; J. P. Blandy personal communication 1988), so its lack of success in some cases is not surprising.

Urethral strictures may be short (arbitrarily defined here, on the basis of the papers quoted below and to allow some degree of comparison, as less than 2 cm), single and situated in the penile urethra. Conversely they may be long (over 2 cm), multiple, situated in the bulbo-membranous urethra and associated with urinary tract infection and local para-urethral infection with abscesses and fistulae. It is therefore not surprising that the results of therapy will vary. It is generally agreed that the short, penile stricture with little periurethral fibrosis

Table 5.1. Review of published results of endoscopic urethrotomy

	Andronaco et al. (1984)	Smith et al. (1983, 1984)	Abdel-Hakim et al. (1983)	Chilton et al. (1983)	Matouschek et al. (1978)	Holm-Neilsen et al. (1984)
No. of patients	100	137	103	412[a]	547	225
Follow-up (yr)[b]	>1	3 (1–7)	>1	1–5	1–6	3–7
Overall cure (%)	62	80[c]	95	50	79	77
Cure after one cut	—	50	49.5	—	—	54
Simple	58/88 (66%)	—	—	—	—	—
Complex	4/12 (33%)	—	—	—	—	—
Av. no. of treatments	—	2.27	1.5	1.8	1.2	1.6

[a]261 patients undergoing urethroplasty and 151 patients undergoing urethrotomy.
[b]Mean or range.
[c]Smith states that "79.6% required no further treatment" but that 44.6% "were cured".

will be treated adequately by any of the available manoeuvres: in particular, good results have been reported for urethrotomy (see Table 5.1).

When studies including a long follow-up period are assessed successful results are in the range 75% at 5 years (Fourcade 1981) to 79% at 5 years in the largest series reported of 547 patients (Matouschek 1978). However, as the data on Table 5.1 show, approximately half of the patients required more than one urethrotomy to relieve their symptoms, i.e. the incidence of recurrence is significant. This is especially true in the "complicated" strictures. Andronaco et al. (1984) reported 100 patients followed up over 1 year. Of these, 88 had short strictures of which 58 (66%) were successfully treated by one endoscopic urethrotomy. However, of the 12 (12%) with long strictures 8 (66%) required further treatment.

Turner-Warwick (1988) has described the complications that may follow the application of what he recognises as "the most valuable procedure available to the general urologist for the resolution of spongio-urethral strictures" including extension of the "spongiofibrosis", sphincter damage, the development of false passages, periurethral pockets and abscess cavities, caverno-fibrotic chordee and meatal distortion (Turner-Warwick 1988). He goes on to question certain practices, particularly the use of the urethrotome simply to cut the fibrotic obstruction resulting from pelvic fracture distraction injuries, which he cautions is not a true stricture and cannot be approached in the same way as the more commonly encountered spongio-urethral stricture since removal of the fibrotic tissue is required rather than simply cutting it.

The results of urethrotomy or dilatation are therefore likely to be related to the length of the stricture and to the degree of periurethral scarring. Whatever treatment is used the recurrence rates in complicated strictures remain disappointing. If the treatment failures and incidence of restricturing are related to the degree of fibrosis then dilatation and urethrotomy cannot be expected to reduce this.

Thus there appears a gap in present treatment: when existing blind or endoscopic methods fail or are not satisfactory and when urethroplasty appears the only alternative. It is in this situation that laser therapy may be advantageous, particularly if it can effect removal of stricture tissue. Laser treatments have heretofore been sporadically reported with surprisingly varied results and with often short follow-up periods.

Laser Treatment of Urethral Strictures

Bulow et al. (1979a, b) described the use of the neodymium yttrium aluminium garnet (YAG) laser on canine and human urethral strictures. The laser was directed down a fibre system using gas cooling and a stream of gas to keep the distal lenses (of both cystoscope and the original, relatively primitive beam delivery channels) free from debris. A series of pulses were fired at the stricture and a 1-cm long stricture is described as requiring 20 minutes to treat. The authors suggested that less of a fibrous response ought to be expected after YAG laser coagulation, resulting in less re-stricturing, and proposed the use of a CO_2 laser as ideal in this respect. Camey and Le Duc (1980) similarly used a YAG laser producing 40–55 W on canine strictures (and prostatic adenomas) and concluded that "tissues were volatilised without bleeding and only moderate heating".

Rothauge (1980) reported the use in 40 patients of an argon laser, which he preferred to the YAG laser owing to the lower depth of penetration of the laser energy. He also stressed that for there to be any advantage over optical urethrotomy the whole of the strictured area should be vaporised rather than using the laser as a urethrotome in one position or even for multiple incisions. The immediate results were good (in terms of flow rates and lack of complications) though in the first year 6 patients required re-treatment. These were described as "early cases before the need for complete removal of the stricture ring" was appreciated. Further follow-up has been reported (Noske et al. 1987) in which brief details of 208 stricture patients were presented. Rothauge's group concluded that the stricture recurrence rate was approximately 30% (or 70% success after one treatment) in previously untreated patients and "almost the rule" for previously treated patients.

Since then most interest has focused on the use of the YAG laser. In 1984 Shanberg et al. reported 6 cases of complicated strictures which had all undergone multiple previous dilatations and optical urethrotomy. The patients underwent laser treatment of their strictures as outpatients, with catheter drainage for 48 hours; in a short (6-month) follow-up period they had no recurrence of their strictures. However, Smith and Dixon (1984) reported that although 17 patients with complicated strictures, all of whom had undergone repeated dilatation and 13 of whom had had previous internal urethrotomy, showed good immediate results after YAG laser treatment, there was a 64% recurrence rate within 6 months. The authors concluded that "with the method described, YAG laser phototherapy appears to offer no treatment advantages over conventional therapy". In their discussion they point out the theoretical advantage of an argon laser in producing more immediate tissue vaporisation than the more deeply penetrating YAG laser, and that based on physical principles a CO_2 laser would be the most promising laser if the problems of lack of a waveguide fibre and the strong absorption of CO_2 laser energy by water (in the irrigation fluid and within the urinary tract) could be overcome.

The technical problems associated with the use of the CO_2 laser should not be underestimated. Because of the intense absorption of CO_2 laser light by water it is necessary for the endoscopy to be performed in a gaseous environment rather than using liquid irrigation, i.e. with insufflation of a gas such as CO_2. As much urine as possible should be removed from the urinary passages being examined. Rendering the urinary tract "dry" enough to use the CO_2 laser effectively is a major challenge. Measures must be taken to prevent the vascular entrapment of large volumes of CO_2 so as to prevent gas embolism. This is particularly likely to happen in the highly vascular urethra, especially if difficult manoeuvres are required as may be the case with complex strictures. However, the major problems involved have not prevented a series of authors from attempting to solve them.

Wilscher et al. (1978) described the development of a CO_2 laser cystoscope, the CO_2 laser energy being transmitted down a rigid but jointed arm which was attached to a large bore (26Fr) endoscope. The laser beam entered the instrument at right angles to the axis of the endoscope and was then directed down its length by reflection off a nickel-plated copper mirror within the endoscope which was also adapted to allow CO_2 gas insufflation. Energy losses were

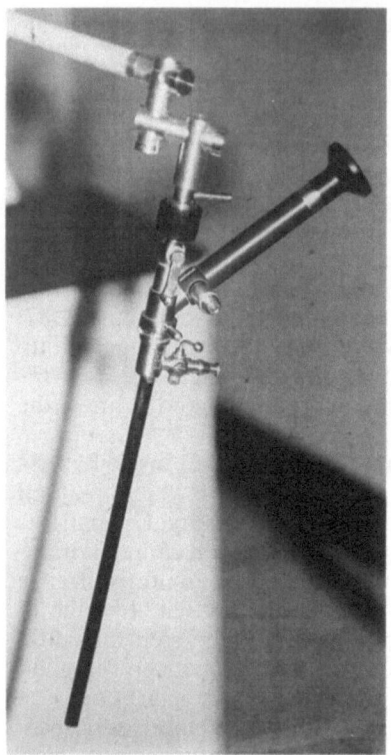

Fig. 5.1. Early prototype clinical laser urethrotome. based on the Storz nephroscope. ready for use.

excessive and use of this prototype difficult. Further developments such as the incorporation of zinc selenide lenses along the laser channel within the instrument made the model smaller and more efficient. with a power of 2–10 W available at the end of the cystoscope. but use remained difficult (Wilscher 1985). Though its effects on dog bladder mucosa are described. the authors were unable to apply this method to urethral strictures.

Bulow and Levene (1979) developed a CO_2 laser endoscope without a mobile arm system and later presented details of a hand-held CO_2 laser connected directly to a cystoscope (Bulow 1984) which appears an attractive proposition – especially with further developments reducing the size of CO_2 lasers.

Sacknoff (1985) described a prototype CO_2 laser cystoscope based on a laparoscope with channels for the fibre-optics. the laser beam. and two for the inflow and outflow of gas. McNicholas and colleagues (1986, 1987) have described the development of a series of relatively slender (18–20Ch) CO_2 laser endoscopes. modified by the Storz company and based on the nephroscope pattern with an offset eyepiece allowing the insertion of disposable rigid or semi-rigid 0.8–3.0-mm diameter waveguides with careful pressure monitoring of the insufflation CO_2 gas and of the intraurethral pressure. Laser pulse durations were 4–6 ms and the peak power at the tip of the endoscope was 5 kW/ cm^2. The CO_2 laser energy is transmitted from the laser to the tip of the endoscope by a series of hollow ceramic waveguides. which have the advan-

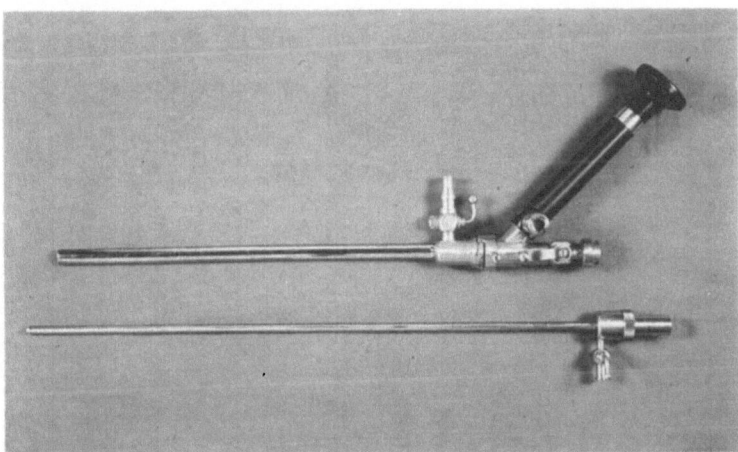

Fig. 5.2. The prototype clinical laser urethrotome, based on the Storz nephroscope, with the wave-guide that can be passed down the operating channel of the endoscope. (Courtesy Institute of Urology.)

tages of being both highly conductive for laser light and cheap. The laser can be focused and defocused to alter the tissue effect by moving the waveguide. Figs. 5.1 and 5.2 show the prototype clinical instrument based on the Storz nephroscope, with the waveguide which can be passed down the operating channel of the endoscope.

The conclusions from the animal experimental work were that CO_2 laser vaporisation of urethral strictures was indeed possible and good healing was found, especially with high powers and with a pulsed-mode laser. This increased peak pulse power by decreasing pulse duration and so appeared to reduce the thermal effect, as was manifest by less charring of tissues (see Fig. 5.3, and Fig. 5.4 opposite p. 90).

The clinical experience in 6 cases (Table 5.2) indicated that the procedure was quick, relatively easy and safe for simple strictures. With follow-up of between 3 and 14 months (mean 6 months) results were at least as good as would be expected from traditional endoscopic urethrotomy but not obviously better – though clearly these are small numbers from which to draw any conclusions.

In our experience it is very easy to lose the true lumen when cutting through complex strictures with the CO_2 laser and gas entrapment is more likely. In addition urethral manipulation can be difficult in these cases and it is almost impossible to keep urine, debris or blood from depositing on the end of the waveguide and the objective lens of the endoscope, thereby reducing laser power and visibility.

The difficulties of CO_2 laser endoscopy of the urinary tract are not to be underestimated. The techniques developed are being taken up by the laser endoscope manufacturers and may be more easily applied to endoscopy of other body cavities where larger-bore endoscopes can be used.

Shanberg et al. (1988) have subsequently described the use of the potassium titanyl phosphate (KTP) laser in 20 patients with 22 urethral strictures. All were failures of previous treatment methods (usually urethrotomy and dilatation).

Table 5.2. CO_2 laser treatment of urethral strictures: clinical results

	FR1	FR2	FR3
Four primary strictures			
3 simple	6	52	42
	17	47	—
	13	44	30
1 complex	3	22	—
Two recurrent strictures			
1 simple	8	49	32
1 complex	8	50	19

FR1. flow rate prior to CO_2 laser urethrotomy.
FR2. flow rate 6 weeks after CO_2 laser urethrotomy.
FR3. flow rate 6 months after CO_2 laser urethrotomy.

The KTP laser gives "CO_2 like" cutting but can be transmitted down a fibre and both passes through and is effective under irrigation fluids. Over the still relatively short follow-up (6–14 months) the authors claim overall success in 68.2% of their patients (success being defined as a twofold increase in the original flow rate or an "open" urethrogram). They also felt the laser would be useful in a range of other open and endoscopic procedures and this laser does appear to be relatively efficient in energy terms.

Techniques of Laser Urethrotomy

Essentially the argon, YAG and KTP lasers are conducted to the site of the stricture via flexible quartz glass fibres passed down any appropriate

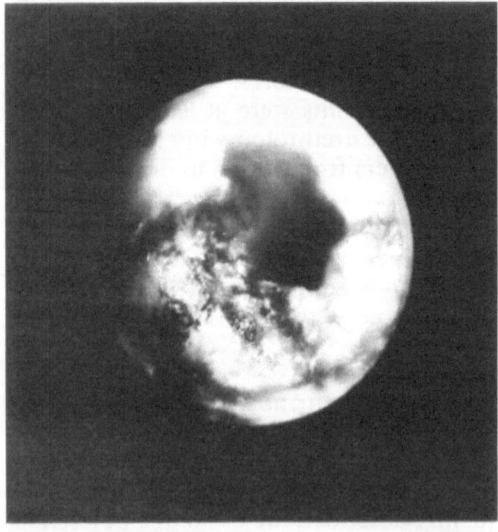

Fig. 5.3. Canine stricture after partial CO_2 laser vaporisation using a continuous wave laser at 10 W, showing excessive charring with reasonable tissue removal.

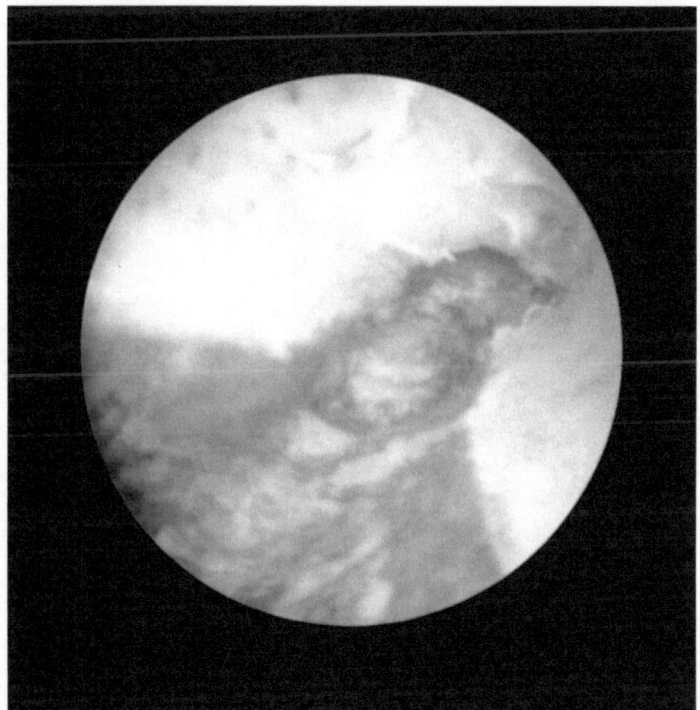

Fig. 5.4. Human stricture after pulsed CO_2 laser urethrotomy using a clinical prototype producing 12–18W average power at a pulse repetition rate of 100 Hz. Increasing peak pulse power by decreasing pulse duration appeared to reduce the thermal effect as was manifest by less charring of tissues. The appearances are of a clean cut through the stricture into the spongiosal tissue.

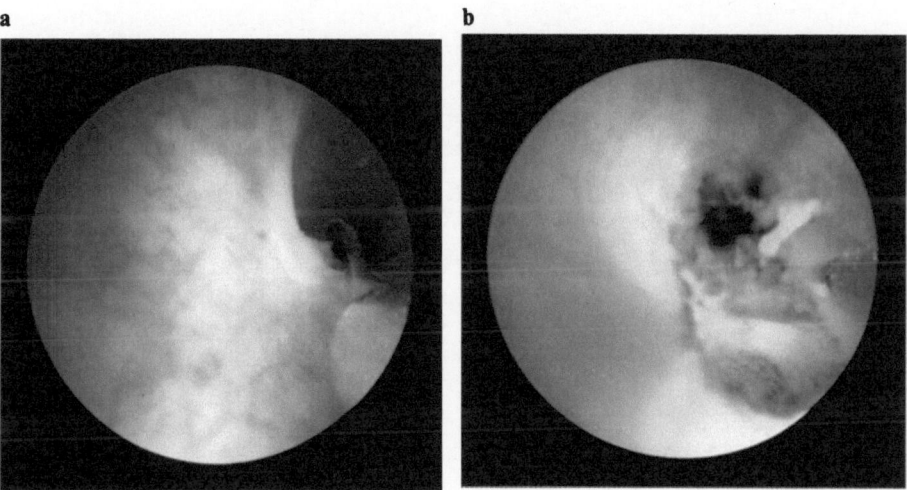

Fig. 5.5. The CO_2 laser waveguide is placed close to the face of the stricture at the 6 o'clock to 7 o'clock position (**a**) and then fired in short bursts (**b**).

Fig. 1.4 Metal surface after pulsed CO_2 laser radiation ... laser irradiation ... metal material ... typical range of 10^{11} ... laser power density ...

endoscope. We have found the Storz urethrotome most suitable; alternatively the newer, smooth-ended, small-bore cystoscopes designed for outpatient cystoscopy can be used. Eye protection is necessary, a suitable protective glass filter eyepiece that clips on over the endoscope eyepiece being ideal.

Endoscopy proceeds as normal until the stricture is seen. The laser fibre is inserted, the laser enabled and the stricture tissue irradiated. The stricture is cut with the "cold knife" urethrotome first, after which the ragged edges of the stricture are coagulated until they shrink and show signs of thermal injury as described by Perez-Castro and Martinez-Pinero (1982). Shanberg et al. (1984) and Smith and Dixon (1984) simply photocoagulated their strictures, following this with dilatation. For the YAG laser a power of 40–50 W for 2–3-second pulses is appropriate, although it is our impression that at the present state of development simple YAG laser treatment of urethral strictures is in fact inappropriate! The early results with the KTP laser are encouraging and the reader is referred to Shanberg et al. (1988) for practical details. In the laboratory it was clear to us that the most obvious difference between the KTP and YAG lasers was that the KTP laser could be drawn over the tissue surface, in direct tissue contact, without unduly damaging the fibre tip. The effect was of a superficial cutting action with a minor degree of coagulation. The KTP can therefore be seen as similar in effect to the CO_2 laser but with the advantage that it is easily transmissible through a standard flexible glass fibre and through urological irrigation fluids.

CO_2 laser urethrotomy is also inappropriate for the general laser user, at least at present. Those experimenting with this method will have found a combination of laser and suitable endoscope that allows reliable endoscopy with gas (invariably CO_2, due to its ready absorption) and will have worked out a method of preventing high pressures being developed in the urethra. The essential details of our method of experimental CO_2 laser urethrotomy are outlined below.

The patient is treated under general anaesthetic in the standard fashion and undergoes routine urethrocystoscopy using liquid irrigation fluids. The patient's end tidal pCO_2 is monitored using a capnograph. It has been suggested that an increase in this value, as a result of vascular entrapment of CO_2, precedes significant clinical signs (Shulman and Aronson 1984). Readings are taken from the screen at 30-second intervals. As part of our experimental studies patients with more complex strictures are monitored even more closely, using a mass spectrometer to analyse biochemical changes in detail.

We use a CO_2 insufflator that can be set so that pressures sensed by a pressure transducer in the equipment will not exceed certain pre-programmed limits. We insufflate at approximately 20 mmHg pressure which allows adequate unfolding and distension of the urethra. A 12–14 gauge plastic cannula is placed in the bladder by suprapubic puncture and left on low-pressure constant suction in an attempt to remove not only all urine from the bas-fond of the bladder but CO_2 gas and smoke in due course.

Once the stricture is seen the laser insert is placed down the instrument channel of the endoscope, brought very close to the surface of the stricture (Fig. 5.5, opposite p.90) and then fired in short bursts a second or so in duration. Aiming specifically at the 6 o'clock to 7 o'clock position of the stricture avoids compromising any reconstructive "roof-strip" procedure that may become necessary. A trench should be cut completely through the stricture and into normal urethra beyond. Once set up the process of CO_2 laser urethrotomy is very quick and frequent positional checks are necessary to avoid cutting too deeply (usually signified by increased bleeding) or cutting away from the correct path of the urethra. The appearance should be of a clean cut through stricture tissue and down to relatively normal spongiosal tissue (for the bulbar and penile urethra) (see Fig. 5.4, opposite p.90). A 14Ch silastic catheter is passed and left for 3 days.

Condylomatous Disease

Introduction

In the UK the treatment of condylomatous disease of the genitalia is usually the preserve of venereologists. Their clinics are at present full of patients presenting with manifestations of infection by the human papilloma virus (HPV). One result of the vast increase in patients with this socially unacceptable and contagious infection is that a proportion of them will develop conditions requiring specialist urological advice and treatment.

In our practice, we see such patients from two major venereology clinics in London. These patients fall into three categories. First, there are those who have disease of the genitalia resistant to the full range of therapeutic options available to the venereologist. Secondly, there are those who have developed complications from traditional treatments, which in most cases means meatal stenosis as a result of the application of podophyllin. Thirdly, there are those whose disease is atypical and involves other parts of the urogenital tract apart from the genital skin. This last group comprises mainly those with disease in the urethral meatus, which is characteristically difficult to eradicate and which acts as a potent reservoir for reinfection both of the patient and of his sexual partners. Finally there is a small sub-group of males whose disease involves not just the meatus but indeed the whole length of the urethra, and these patients certainly need expert urological advice.

The disease is irritating, offensive and unsightly, but its real significance is in the relationship of HPV infection to the subsequent development of squamous cancers. The link between some types of HPV infection (16, 18, 31, 33, 35) and subsequent cervical neoplasia is becoming stronger (Crum et al. 1983) and it is now clear that the female consorts of males with penile condylomata acuminata are at increased risk of cervical neoplasia (Campion et al. 1985). A recent British study of females under 20 years of age referred for colposcopy found that of 38 with external genital warts 26 (68%) had histologically proven cervical intra-epithelial neoplasia (Haddad et al. 1988).

The role of laser treatment in the disease is in the management of those with extensive resistant disease, those with urethral meatal warts and those with urethral viral tumours. It is essential for the urologist to have a close working relationship with expert venereological colleagues.

The proponents of laser treatment of viral wart diseases of the genitalia fall into two groups: those who champion the use of the CO_2 laser (Baggish 1985; Rosemberg 1985) and those who describe the benefits of using the YAG laser. We have used both and in general terms either can be very effective; to a certain extent the choice of laser will be dictated by what is available. Gynaecologists will be more familiar with the CO_2 laser and will almost certainly have such a laser fitted to a colposcope. Urologists, with less need of the particular characteristics of the CO_2 laser and greater familiarity with the YAG laser tend to choose it in preference to the CO_2 laser. However, whilst admitting our choice may be largely due to convenience, we do prefer the YAG laser, which we have found to be well tolerated by most of our patients.

Laser Treatment of Genital Wart Disease

We take a full sexual history and enquire into the general health of the patient. Sexual orientation of the patient should be determined and human immunodeficiency virus (HIV) testing done if necessary and according to local practices.

We explain the method of treatment to the patient, how it will be performed, the possible complications and whatever discomfort may be experienced subsequently. This is also a good time to explain how and where further treatment will be performed, should it be needed. In our unit we explain to the patients that there is no guarantee the treatment they are about to receive will destroy all disease, since there may be areas of subclinical viral infection not revealed during the examination which will obviously not be treated and may therefore act as the source of further infection. The patient is also instructed to use a condom to protect his partner during the ensuing 3 months and is advised that his partner, if female, should seek examination to ensure she has no cervical abnormalities.

Throughout the following discussion the term "he" is used in referring to patients since most of our practice relates to the treatment of males. We have a small number of female patients who have had extensive condylomatous disease of the vulva treated, but this has generally been complicated by a marked degree of discomfort after treatment. Until we have developed further methods of overcoming these symptoms in conjunction with our gynaecological and venereological colleagues, we are restricting our treatment to males. In view of the potentially serious risk of developing squamous cancers of the cervix and vulva, we feel female cases should be under the overall care of a gynaecologist.

For those males with very extensive disease a general anaesthetic is often used, though a local ringblock at the base of the penis with lignocaine (lidocaine) will often allow treatment of fairly extensive lesions on the penis. The development of "eutectic" mixtures of the local anaesthetic agents lignocaine and prilocaine (EMLA, Astra Pharmaceuticals) has opened up the prospect of effective surface anaesthesia of the skin without the need for injecting anaesthetic agents. In the UK the manufacturing company do not have a product licence as yet for this application of EMLA, but there has been increasing experience of its use in Scandinavia and our early experience on a trial basis has been encouraging.

The EMLA cream is applied liberally over the penile skin approximately 1 hour before treatment, and a condom put on to keep the cream from being wiped off. Even if complete anaesthesia is not achieved, it allows the easy injection of lignocaine to supplement anaesthesia if necessary. For those patients with a few relatively small lesions, direct injection of local anaesthetic under the lesion through a 21 gauge needle is the simplest and quickest method.

If the YAG laser is being used the fibre should be cooled, so the traditional type of fibre as used by gastroenterologists or pulmonary specialists is needed. This consists of the same 400-μm or 600-μm quartz glass fibre but with a heavy plastic "cannula" lying loosely around it. The cannula is manufactured in such a way that when the laser is fired, a jet of cooling gas (usually air) is directed down it to cool the fibre tip.

With the patient in an appropriate position, the genitalia are inspected using a good light. The use of a hand-held lens or a colposcope if available is helpful and the penis is then liberally doused in a 3%–5% solution of acetic acid. This so-called aceto-white test tends to show up abnormal areas of epithelium as white patches, particularly those areas of hyperplastic or dysplastic epithelium where viral activity is present. Obviously macroscopic lesions should turn white, but in addition to these, other areas may also reveal themselves as areas of abnormal epithelium. In an awake patient the acetic acid can be quite irritating, particularly if left for a long time and certainly if it spills onto the skin of the scrotum. The patient's confidence is usually markedly diminished at this point, and certainly his cooperation! It is therefore worth avoiding spilling acetic acid on the scrotum and being prepared to wash off the acid with liberal quantities of saline once the abnormal areas have been identified.

We use the laser at a power of between 15 and 20 W and set the pulse duration at 2 seconds. This is a safeguard, and with increasing experience the pulse duration can be set much longer, the actual length of the laser pulses being determined by use of the foot pedal whilst being guided by the visible changes of the irradiated skin. It is of course essential that everyone in the operating room, including the patient, wears appropriate YAG light protecting goggles or glasses.

Treatment consists simply of bringing the fibre close to the areas of abnormal skin and firing the laser. We have found no advantage in the focusing handpieces available, preferring to increase or decrease the power density and the tissue effects by moving the fibre closer or further away. However, if the skin has become dry there is often a very brisk skin response as the target skin is rapidly heated and it may disrupt in the target zone ("popcorning": S. G. Lundquist, personal communication 1986) due to steam formation. In our experience this tends to cause delayed healing and more discomfort subsequently, so skin being treated is kept moist by irrigation with cold saline, which can be dropped onto the target area from a sponge or syringe. This method should also prevent the burning of skin and the release of any plume of smoke, thereby avoiding any possible risk of the transmission of viable viral material (T. Malloy, personal communication 1989).

Adequate laser treatment is manifest by changes similar to those seen in endoscopic laser practice, i.e. the target tissue shrinks and tends to rise up and become white. Further coagulation is not necessary and once all visible lesions and all areas of abnormal epithelium have been treated the treatment is complete. The patient is warned that these areas will tend to slough off over the next week to 10 days and is encouraged to take daily salt baths. The remaining raw areas may take several weeks to heal completely. It has impressed us how painless the post-operative course after YAG laser coagulation has been. Obviously, it is important to leave an adequate amount of skin between areas of laser coagulation to allow healing and to avoid any cicatricial contraction.

Laser Treatment of Meatal Disease

The aceto-white test may well show up abnormalities of the urethral meatus. However, since this area may act as a reservoir for recurrent infections it is vital that any HPV infection here is not overlooked and careful inspection is essential. In practice it is often difficult to inspect the whole meatal area and all the recesses of the fossa navicularis. Indeed this area may be the last remaining blind spot in the urinary tract! Pulling the edges of the meatus apart may reveal something of the interior and the use of a speculum such as a nasal speculum or urethroplasty speculum may well help. However, we have found an otoscope (Keeler Ltd.) with a modified nozzle and the addition of air insufflation to be an excellent means of inspecting the distal 2 or 3 cm of the male urethra with good illumination and distension of the lumen (Figs. 5.6–5.8). The use of this instrument, which we have christened the meatoscope, has helped ensure that small lesions in this vital area are not missed, and its use has been enthusiastically taken up in our associated venereology clinics (R. N. Thin, personal communication 1989).

Patients are reviewed at 1 week and at 6 weeks and finally at 3 and 6 months. Obviously in less academic practice there is less need for this number of reviews.

We have treated 26 men referred with resistant condyloma, of whom 4 had a degree of meatal stenosis from their previous treatment and 3 had total urethral involvement by masses of wart tissue (Fig. 5.9). There has been one recurrence on follow-up, which is likely to have been due to undertreatment of subclinical lesions on the penile shaft.

The 3 patients with urethral tumours underwent initial endoscopic mapping of their lesions and biopsy. The tumours characteristically stop at the distal sphincter and once biopsied a "test area" is lasered at 15–20 W in 2-second

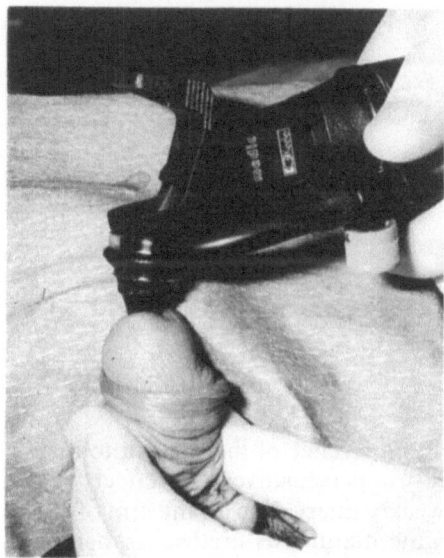

Fig. 5.6. The meatoscope.

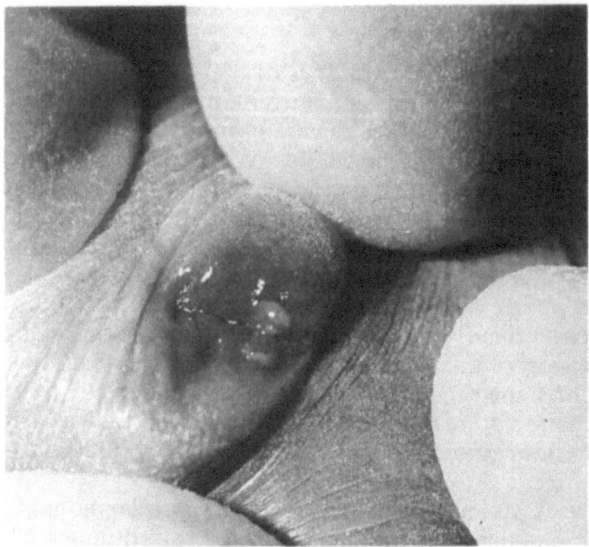

Fig. 5.7. Meatal wart prior to treatment.

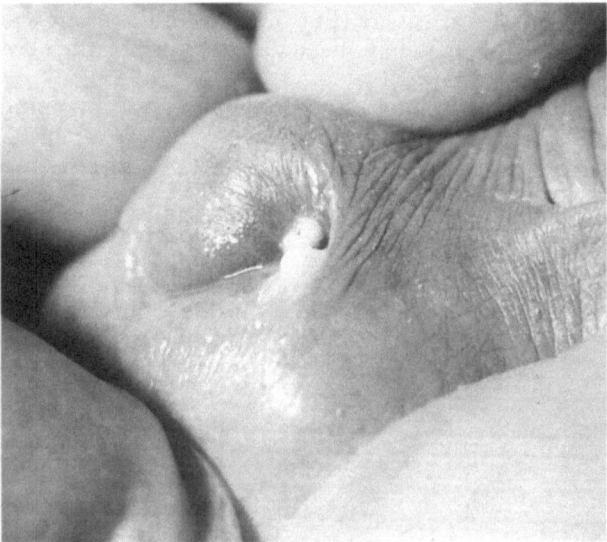

Fig. 5.8. Coagulated meatal wart.

bursts over a 2-cm length of the whole circumference of the urethra to assess whether or not the urethra will prove unduly hypersensitive to the effects of the YAG laser. The patient is re-treated at 6-weekly intervals, with the aim of coagulating all visible lesions in much the same manner as urethral transitional cell cancer is treated (Fig. 5.10). Two patients have been clear of disease for over 18 months and one is about to receive his third treatment.

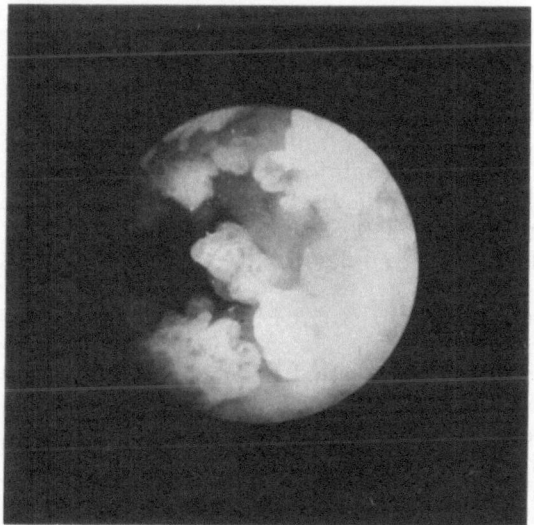

Fig. 5.9. Multiple urethral condylomata.

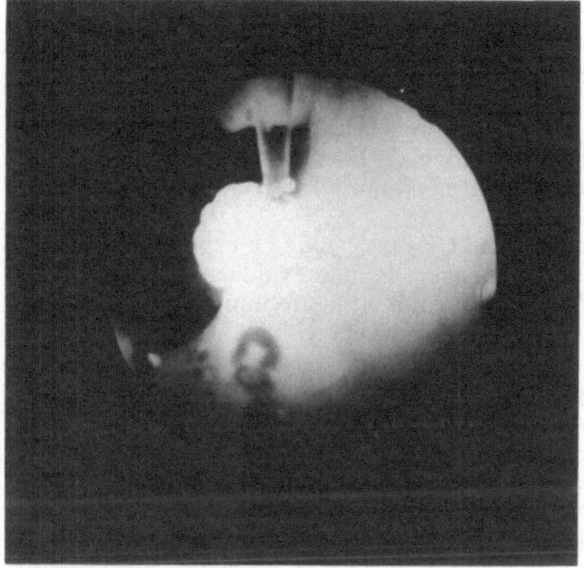

Fig. 5.10. YAG laser coagulation of urethral condylomata.

Use of the CO_2 Laser

The largest experience reported to date in laser treatment of condylomata acuminata is with the CO_2 laser. One advantage of the CO_2 laser is that it may well be available in an environment where the treatment of cervical abnormalities with the aid of a colposcope is established. The combination of CO_2 laser and colposcope allows examination of the target organ under good illumination and magnification and accurate direction of the laser beam (usually by means of a "joystick" micromanipulator on the colposcope) to burn off the areas of abnormal epithelium as indicated by the white changes of the aceto-white test. However, treatment is usually straightforward in most instances even if such equipment is not available, particularly as very portable and hand-held small CO_2 lasers are becoming available. Power levels from 2 to 10 W are sufficient and the beam can be focused and defocused to alter the relative cutting or haemostatic effects of the laser.

Local infiltration with 1% lidocaine (lignocaine) or EMLA cream provides sufficient analgesia for the treatment of small penile condylomata but extensive penile or perianal lesions may require regional or general anaesthesia (Lundquist and Lindstedt 1983; Rosemberg 1985). For small lesions a setting of 2–10 W on a continuous wave mode is sufficient because vaporisation proceeds rapidly. Larger lesions may require a higher output (20–30 W) and the process is helped by repeatedly wiping the surface clear of charred tissue to expose deeper layers for treatment. There is, however, more burning and a certain amount of smoke generation which is not to be encouraged.

Treatment in general terms follows the same pattern as described above (Meandzija 1985; Rosemberg 1985). The operator's eyes are protected by the colposcope. If the colposcope is not being used then all staff present, including the operator, must wear protective eyewear. Clear plastic glasses or goggles or one's own personal spectacles with sideguards are suitable. Under good magnification the superficial layers of the penile skin and/or vulval skin and mucous membrane can be destroyed and good, rapid healing of the laser-coagulated areas expected. Lundquist and Lindstedt (1983) described a 95% cure rate in their patients treated with CO_2 laser therapy (mainly) with a follow-up of over 6 months.

The more superficial effect from the CO_2 laser may be expected to lead to quicker healing and less scarring, but there is little evidence that the deeper coagulation resulting from YAG laser treatment is any more damaging. The temptation to destroy larger areas of skin surface with the CO_2 laser on the basis that the tissues will heal satisfactorily is to be avoided.

Riva et al. (1989), in a study to determine whether the CO_2 laser could eradicate widespread subclinical papillomavirus infection, attempted to vaporise the epithelium of the entire female lower genital tract. Post-operative morbidity was considerable and biopsies showed persistence of papillomavirus infection in 88% at follow-up. This would fit with our clinical impression that a widespread viral infection is impossible to eradicate with a focal treatment method. The dangers of thermally damaging a large surface area of epithelium should not be underestimated, and healthy "skin bridges" should be preserved between areas of laser coagulation.

Urethral Haemangiomas

Introduction

Haemangiomas of the penis and particularly those that form in the urethra are very rare (Senoh et al. 1981). True haemangiomas are unrelated to trauma and should be differentiated from arteriovenous (AV) malformations. Unlike AV malformations haemangiomas are not amenable to embolisation. They can present at any age and particularly cause problems during puberty and in adult life after the onset of erections.

Treatment options range from judicious non-interference if they are minor and asymptomatic through local treatment such as diathermy (which is usually unsuccessful) to open surgical procedures involving exposing the bleeding area for oversewing and then repairing the defect. The final option is total urethral excision as described by Tilak (1967).

Before these patients come to final definitive surgery, though, it is worth a trial of endoscopic laser coagulation therapy for a urethral haemangioma. The argon laser is theoretically ideally suited to the coagulation of a blood-filled, thin-walled vessel, and if one is available it should be tried. Unfortunately an argon laser is only likely to be available if the unit concerned has an interest in photodynamic therapy and has been using the argon laser as part of their photodynamic studies. The limited role of the argon laser in mainstream urology has meant that the YAG laser has supplanted it in those urological units equipped with a laser for endoscopic surgery.

In realistic terms the urologist will have to consider the use of a YAG laser and it should be remembered that the reaction of the haemangiomatous urethra is likely to be different from that of any other tissue the laser urologist may have encountered. In addition a quite different effect is required from the laser itself. In most other circumstances, although the laser user desires coagulation, this is preferably not to the extent of causing fibrosis and scarring. For example, whilst treatment of urethral tumours should be effective and complete it should spare the urethra and avoid stricturing if possible. In the treatment of urethral haemangiomas, however, YAG lasers are used to cause a vessel coagulating effect followed, ideally, by the development of a relatively dense subepithelial fibrotic reaction. The end result is in theory a more resistant urethral lining which will act as a barrier against vessel regrowth into the urethral lumen.

Vessels elsewhere in the penis may well bleed, particularly when exposed to trauma, but this generally has a self-limiting effect as the intrapenile pressure increases, eventually tamponading the bleeding point. However, when there is free bleeding from a large-volume, thin-walled, low-pressure vessel into the urethra this tamponading effect is lost and major haemorrhage can result.

Urethral haemangioma is a very unusual condition and there is very little in the laser literature to guide the operator. Smith and Dixon (1984) described 4 cases of bladder haemangioma, 3 treated by the argon laser and 1 by a combination of YAG and argon lasering. Amagai et al. (1981) reported on 5 cases of urethral haemangioma treated by laser: 2 with a CO_2 laser, 2 with an argon laser and 1 with a YAG laser. Very few operative details were given, and little indication as to which of the three lasers used was best in the authors' experience.

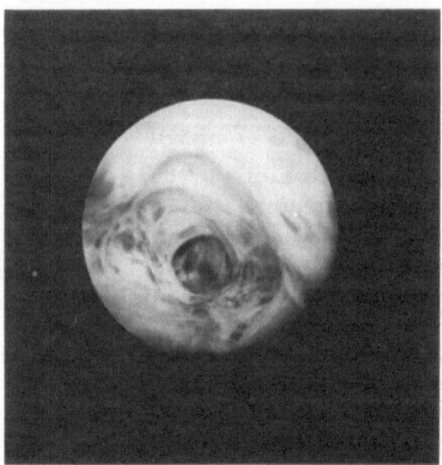

Fig. 5.11. Very extensive penile urethral haemangiomas in a young male.

We cannot see that the CO_2 laser would have a role to play in such a condition. For the reasons outlined above, in practice the YAG laser is the instrument of choice.

Our laser practice includes two young men with very extensive penile haemangiomas (Fig. 5.11). Both presented with frequent, recurrent urethral haemorrhage requiring hospital admission and blood transfusions. In both cases the haemangiomas involve the whole length of the urethra and also involve the pelvis.

Laser Treatment of Urethral Haemangioma

As with all laser coagulation in the urethra the procedure starts with a careful endoscopy and mapping of the anatomical features of the urethra. Great gentleness and care is absolutely essential, because heavy bleeding can occur quite easily. We recommend the use of the 20Ch urethrotome with a 0° viewing telescope. If the urethral lumen is tight on that endoscope then a smaller-bore instrument should be used. The latest generation of smooth-contoured endoscopes designed for outpatient endoscopy are less traumatic than the traditional cystoscope and have the advantage that any instrument passed down their instrument channel, including the laser fibre, will enter directly into the operator's visual field as it leaves the channel (Miller et al. 1987). This greatly reduces the chances of an instrument inadvertently damaging the urethral lining as it leaves the instrument channel.

A suitable area of haemangiomatous urethra is then chosen, the laser enabled and the fibre passed down the chosen endoscope. A low power setting (approximately 10 W) should be used initially and very short pulses of less than half a second. It needs to be judged by watching the effect of the first few pulses on the lining of the urethra whether the duration of the pulses and indeed even the power level can be judiciously increased. At urethral endoscopy a "test strip" is chosen and coagulated, aiming to treat a full circumference of the urethra at the chosen point. This should be near a visible land-mark to enable it to be found at the next treatment 6–8 weeks later.

Care should be taken during this first treatment not to puncture the thin-walled, friable vascular spaces by too vigorous a treatment. Should bleeding occur then catheterisation may be required both to avoid retention of urine and also to help tamponade the bleeding area. A period of pressure over the point of bleeding, particularly if this occurs in the penile urethra, may serve to stop the bleeding.

At the subsequent treatment the test area is assessed and further treatment given if there are no untoward sequelae. An area of rather paler mucosa should be seen in the test area. Treatment then slowly and steadily progresses both downstream and upstream from the test area. A course of the treatments is usually required, but after several visits the operator may be greeted with an encouragingly paler urethral lining. It is of some help to photograph the appearances or better still to record the initial procedure on videotape for com-parison with later appearances.

One of our patients with urethral haemangioma is in the early stages of treat-ment, but the other, a 15-year-old male, had five treatments from October 1987 to mid 1988. During that period the distal penile urethra became much less vascular and his urethral bleeding has ceased for over 6 months. He has had one intercurrent major bleed but this occurred into the para-urethral tissues rather than bursting through into the urethral lumen itself. He had a sausage-shaped swelling surrounding the mid part of his penile urethra due to a tense collection of blood, but this was treated conservatively and has resolved. There has been no effect on his erectile function and it would appear that the bleed-ing was limited to his corpus spongiosum, in which case our therapy may well have achieved its aim of creating a rather more dense urethral lining resistant to the development of blood vessels and thereby reduced the potential for major urethral bleeding.

Tissue Anastomosis and Repair
With S. Flemming

Introduction

The accurate apposition and anastomosis of small tubular structures remains a surgical challenge. The development of microsurgical techniques, particu-larly the development of the operating microscope and fine suture material, has allowed the rapid expansion of plastic surgical reconstruction procedures based on vascularised flaps. The flap may either be on a long vascular pedicle from its site of origin or have its vessels anastomosed to locally situated feeding and draining vessels. Although generally used for plastic surgery these tech-niques have applications in most surgical specialities. The use of magnifica-tion is required to allow the accurate anastomosis of such small structures.

Despite the steady advances in suturing methods and materials there is a long history of attempts to develop alternative techniques avoiding the need for sutures. The principle of non-suture anastomosis of blood vessels was developed by Payr in 1900, tested by Hopfner (1903) and applied clinically by Lexer in 1907. Blakemore et al. (1942, 1943) employed a method using vitallium rings lined with vein grafts. Despite initial success there were problems with application of these techniques and suturing remained the preferred method of anastomosis.

In 1956, Androsov described the use of a staple gun that could be used to join vessels as small as 1.3 mm in diameter; it was adapted by Inokuchi (1961) to perform end-to-side anastomoses. In the late 1950s and early 1960s a variety of non-suture methods were introduced that used cuffs (Carter and Roth 1958) or interlocking rings (Nakayama et al. 1963), but most were either too bulky and cumbersome to use or too rigid to allow expansion of the vessel (Cobett 1967).

Despite some early successes suturing small vessels the major problem then was the quality of suture materials and instruments. Research in microvascular surgery resulted in the development of fine surgical instruments and fine, relatively non-reactive suture materials which replaced earlier larger, more reactive sutures. Concurrent progress in operating microscopes now made anastomosis of vessels as small as 0.2 mm in diameter possible (Huang et al. 1982).

However, all suture material causes some reaction, and this may be a relatively important factor in the patency and healing of these fine anastomoses. New ways of joining tissues that are suitable for use under magnification are therefore always being sought. Most work has been done on microvascular anastomoses and a range of devices incorporating Teflon, tantalum, polythene rings or pinning devices have been tried experimentally without clinical success.

Interest has now turned to tissue glues. Initially cyanoacrylate glues were investigated (Hosbein and Blumenstock 1964) but their exothermic reaction tends to disrupt anastomosis as a result of gas formation, even though they may be useful for bonding flat layers together (Goetz et al. 1966). More recently fibrin polymer glues have shown some promising features (Luke et al. 1986), though further development awaits a method of preparation avoiding any risk of transmission of blood-borne virus particles, especially the human immunodeficiency virus (HIV).

Modern small-calibre anastomotic techniques require the use of magnification. This may be by means of binocular loupes worn on the surgeon's head like spectacles or by the use of an operating microscope. Loupes are relatively cheap and give magnifications between 2 times ($\times 2$) and $\times 10$, although $\times 6$ is generally found to be the maximal comfortable magnification. The disadvantages are the small field of view and small depth of focus, so that minor movements of the surgeon's head will cause the subject to become blurred. Thus the surgeon's head must remain fairly still and this tends to increase fatigue.

The operating microscope gives magnifications between $\times 6$ and $\times 40$ on most commonly used instruments. Field illumination is excellent and the more advanced microscopes allow "zooming" between different magnifications. The surgeon can move about more although, generally, looking away from the site of operation and changing one's point of focus is inefficient and a source of strain. One enormous advantage is that modern microscopes have facilities to allow the assistant and scrub nurse to see exactly what the surgeon is doing, which enables them to help him. Indeed by using the video camera link the rest of the theatre staff can be involved in what may otherwise be a prolonged and rather boring process for them.

Vasectomy and Vasal Re-anastomosis

The presence of an obstructed vas with an apparently normal testicle was described by William Hunter in the eighteenth century. Interest in performing vasectomy developed from Guyon's (1883) postulate that the procedure would lead to prostatic atrophy and would therefore provide a treatment for prostatic obstruction. As a tribute to man's ability to see both sides of a question is it notable that while Sharp in 1909 advocated vasectomy as a means of decreasing sexual aggressiveness, initially in the treatment of a young man guilty of "excessive masturbation" and then for assorted criminals, Steinack in 1918 (Kuss and Gregoire 1988) was later performing the same procedure in an attempt to increase potency!

Proust in 1904 (Murphy 1972) recommended vasectomy for the prevention of epididymo-orchitis following prostatic surgery and the procedure was commonly practised until the advent of appropriate antibacterial therapy. However, its most common indication is the need to reduce male fertility as part of contraceptive efforts. The World Health Organisation estimated in 1981 that some 40 million procedures had been performed. Vasectomy is the fourth commonest surgical procedure in the USA, with approximately 500 000 operations yearly. With modern trends of divorce and remarriage and with the possibility of disaster striking the completed, planned family so that restoration of fertility is desired, it is not surprising that there is a vigorous and rising demand for reversal of vasectomy. Finally there remains a small group of males with primary obstructive azoospermia or oligozoospermia as a result of vasal abnormalities who require reconstruction of the vasa.

Vasectomy reversal was not a frequent operation until recently, however. In 1948 O'Conor sent a questionnaire to American urologists. Of 750 responses only 135 surgeons had performed the operation once or more, giving a total of 450 cases in all with a claimed patency of 42%. Derrick et al. (1973) updated this study by a similar questionnaire to members of the American Urological Association, finding that 542 members had between them performed only 1630 vasovasostomies (VV) with a 38% patency rate and fertility proven by pregnancy of 19.5%. Since then the demand has risen remorselessly, increasing at a steady 0.5%–3% of the rising rate of vasectomies. Rosemberg et al. (1985) have postulated a potential case load for reversal of 30%–50% of all vasectomies if divorce and remarriage rates within the general population are extrapolated to the vasectomised population.

The methods used for VV fall into three main groups:

1. *A macroscopic method.* A fairly simple technique using a small number of relatively large sutures (generally 6.0 nylon, Prolene or Dexon) is most commonly employed in the UK. A stent may or may not be used over which the anastomosis is fashioned and which is removed several days later.

2. *Moderate non-microscopic magnification.* A method using magnification is less common but increasing in popularity. Mostly this will involve the use of ×4 to ×8 magnification binocular loupes and a one- or two-layer anastomosis using 6.0 or possibly even finer (10.0) sutures.

3. *Re-anastomosis by a fully microscopic technique (MSVV).* A fully fledged microscopic technique is used by a few surgeons in the UK but much more frequently in the USA and Western Europe. Characteristically magnification

varies between ×6 and ×20 for various stages of the anastomosis. Fine 10.0 sutures are commonly employed especially if vasoepididymostomy is performed (Silber 1984). The anastomosis itself may be performed in one layer of "all layers" sutures, as a two-layer anastomosis of mucosal and sero-muscular layers (M. Royle, personal communication 1986), or as a combination of mucosal sutures and full-thickness sutures.

Careful, accurate mucosal apposition would seem a prerequisite for a good result as in any other tubular structure (viz. gut and vessels). Success rates are a hotly debated topic. Success can be measured in terms of patency rates implied by the presence of sperm in the ejaculate at a later stage. Contrast patency studies after operation are generally only performed to pinpoint reasons for failure and to confirm the site of problems once failure of sperm to appear in the ejaculate has been established. Thus just how good an anastomosis has been achieved is difficult to assess – only whether sperms are getting across the join. This is, it could be argued, a fairly academic point but it may take some time for a pregnancy to be achieved and a poor join may only allow sperm passage temporarily before stenosing and/or obstructing again or may cause the sperm to be effete and ineffective even when they do manage to cross an unsatisfactory join. Overall, however, the pregnancy rate over 2 years from operation remains the gold standard for assessment of results.

Cos et al. (1983), reviewing published reports of 493 VVs done by 19 surgeons with six different techniques between 1978 and 1983, described an overall patency rate of 81.5% with an overall pregnancy rate of 53.5%. The best patency rates (approximately 90%) were reported by those using a two-layer unstented MSVV method but there was little difference in pregnancy rates (56%–62%) between MSVV and an anastomosis performed using loupe magnification with or without stenting. However, pregnancy rates in those VVs performed "macroscopically" were lower, at 41%–44%.

Certain principal requirements have become clear:

1. A leakproof anastomosis: Hagan and Coffey (1977) showed the damaging effects of any sperm leak at the anastomosis.
2. The preservation of the perivasal adventitia: this requires careful dissection and preservation of tissue vascularity.
3. The avoidance of tension at the anastomotic site.

The proponents, such as Silber (1984), of a purely microsurgical technique, particularly a two-layer method, claim these requirements are ensured and result in pregnancy rates as high as 82%. Similar figures are claimed by exponents of methods using the microscope but performing a modified (and less time-consuming) two-layer anastomosis (Sharlip 1981) and by those advocating loupe magnification, and also simple suture in one layer. Better results might on the whole be expected if the surgeon is experienced and can use an operating microscope and is prepared to spend 2–3 hours meticulously rejoining the vas in two careful layers. This method has become popular in North American urological practice and microsurgery has become a part of the urologist's training. However, not everyone has the time and/or the inclination to spend so long on this procedure. If a method could be found that was faster, might improve efficacy and could reduce the amount of foreign material implanted then that method should be assessed carefully.

One of the major characteristics of laser light is that it can be sharply focused. It can also cause a relatively precise thermal action of a degree and depth that can be altered according to the choice of laser and the wavelength, the duration of the exposure and the power density (W/cm^2). It is therefore not surprising that this finely tunable tool has been considered as a tissue welder.

Laser Tissue Welding

The principle of tissue welding is that the approximated tissue surfaces can be heated to the point where they will stick together. This principle was applied by Sigel and co-workers (Que and Sigel 1965) who used electrocautery to anastomose vessels successfully in experimental animals, but the bond was not reliable in arteries. The major problems were delivering the correct amount of energy to form a weld, and preventing the diathermy forceps from sticking to the tissues so that the bond was not damaged when they were removed.

The advantages that lasers have over this method are that defined amounts of energy can be delivered and that because the energy (or heat) source is remote it does not come into direct contact with the tissues to be joined.

Laser welding has the attraction that the low-power systems required are moderately cheap and can be relatively easily attached to operating microscopes, from where the beam can be conducted on to the operating field of view. The beam can be positioned precisely in the operative field, usually by means of a finger-controlled "joystick" on the microscope, so lends itself to use for fine microscopic procedures as spot size can be made as small or as large as necessary by optical manipulation (within the microscope).

A laser welding method might:

1. Allow precise coagulation and welding of small-calibre tubes with less damaging manipulation of delicate tissues.
2. Reduce or avoid the need for suture material and thus reduce the inflammatory stimulus and foreign body reaction that sutures cause.
3. Thereby reduce the most common cause of technical errors: the inaccurate placement of sutures (Lidman and Daniel 1981).
4. Create a more "leakproof" join since a complete "welding" ring would be created and there would be fewer holes caused by the traumatic passage of needles and sutures.

As described earlier the absorption and transmission of light in tissues will depend on the wavelength of the incident light, and the absorption and scattering characteristics of the tissues at that wavelength. All three common continuous wave lasers have been used for laser tissue welding, but from what has been said in earlier chapters it is likely that the CO_2 laser will produce a very superficial weld, with the least damage to the surrounding tissues, while the argon and YAG lasers will probably produce deeper welds. Urological research has tended strongly towards the CO_2 laser, but it is fair to say that the most appropriate laser has not been defined and realistically no one laser or set of laser parameters is likely to weld all structures equally well.

Both YAG and argon laser light are far more dependent upon the optical properties of the tissue upon which they are incident than CO_2 laser light because of the latter's strong absorption in water. The modified 1326-nm wave-length YAG laser has been claimed by some to be much more suitable for thicker welds than the more commonly used 1064-nm wavelength YAG light (Dew 1986). Confusion arises since transmission studies indicate that 1326-nm radiation is absorbed better by water and it would therefore be expected to pene-trate less than 1064-nm light!

The first use of lasers in vascular surgery was reported by Yahr and Strully (1967); they used a CO_2 laser. Klink et al. (1978) used a low-power CO_2 laser to seal fallopian tubes and Jain and Gorish (1979) used a continuous wave YAG laser to seal tears made in small blood vessels. Jain (1983) developed the tech-nique further to perform end-to-end and end-to-side anastomoses. His results encouraged a great deal of further work in many plastic surgical centres. Others have reported the use of the argon (Kreuger and Almquist 1985) and more commonly the CO_2 laser (Neblett et al. 1986) to achieve "welding", usually reporting work on blood vessels.

All of the possible advantages outlined above apply to the re-anastomosis of the vas, where the development of sperm granulomas as a result of sperm leak through the vasal suture line (or indeed through the puncture holes made by relatively large-calibre needles and suture material) may give rise to an obstructing mass which reduces patency (Hagan and Coffey 1977). Sperm leak, by allowing exposure of a large quantity of sperms to the circulatory system, also has immunological consequences (antibody formation) that may reduce fertility even if a reasonable number of sperms appear in the ejaculate. It has been suggested that tissue welding using a laser might produce a watertight or, more accurately, a sperm-tight seal more quickly and more easily than MSVV.

In the first reported work on laser welding of the vas Morris modified the technique used for vessel anastomosis using a 500-μm spot size, a power of 200 mW and exposure times of 0.05 seconds (Lynne et al. 1983). Dew and asso-ciates (Dew et al. 1983; Dew 1983, 1986) used CO_2, argon and YAG lasers of two different wavelengths to weld the vas deferens as well as blood vessels, skin and nerves. Dew (1984) described his experience of CO_2 welding of a range of soft tissues including the vas: he found superior wound healing, possibly due to less surgical manipulation, less foreign material and a less technically demanding procedure. Rosemberg et al. (1985) reported a welded anastomosis of the vas in three acutely divided dog vasa using a large spot size (2 mm), a power of 1.8 W and an exposure of 0.2 seconds (i.e. a power density of approxi-mately 45 W/cm^2).

Jarow et al. (1986), with a method similar to the one used in our studies (and described below), anastomosed human vasa in vitro and rat vasa in vivo using a welding technique with a milliwatt CO_2 laser. They found that the incidence of sperm granuloma was unacceptably high, although patency was almost as good as for sutured anastomoses. Sperm granulomas were more common in the welded anastomoses. These authors found that bursting pressures were much higher for laser-anastomosed vessels than for sutured vessels, while longi-tudinal strength was greater for the sutured anastomoses. McNicholas et al. (1986, 1987) reported their experience of welding the previously obstructed and unobstructed rabbit vas. In these studies the bursting pressures were not higher in the laser-assisted group immediately after anastomosis – indeed the oppo-site was true. At later stages the lasered and sutured groups had similar burst-ing pressures. Sperm granulomas were not found as commonly. Stein and

Cooley (1988), using a similar milliwatt CO_2 laser to weld rat vasa in two layers, also found the incidence of sperm granulomas to be low and equal to that occurring in the microsurgical group.

Rosemberg et al. (1988) performed laser-assisted vasovasostomies with a microsurgical CO_2 laser at a range of powers varying from 50 mW through 80 mW and to 100 mW (and thereby giving power densities of 20, 32 and 40 W/cm²). There were many leaks at 50 mW and 80 mW but a good welded join at 100 mW, i.e. this study suggests the need for a power density of 40 W/cm² or above to achieve a strong bond. Rosemberg in 1987 described clinical laser-assisted vasovasostomy; he was closely followed by Shanberg's group (A. Shanberg, personal communication 1989).

The characteristic features of the studies of laser welding of the vas mentioned above are firstly that the anastomoses were in fact "laser assisted", and secondly that they were performed on vasa that had only just been divided, thus avoiding one of the common surgical problems of this procedure: how to re-appose accurately tubular structures the calibre of one end of which is greatly enlarged due to obstructive changes to the other end which, being empty, has tended to shrink.

Belker (1985) suggested that proper comparison of the laser and traditional techniques can only be made if the experimental subjects have been vasectomised some time prior to re-anastomosis so that there is disparity in size between the ends to be re-anastomosed, as is found in the clinical case. Our studies were designed to incorporate these factors. Good welding in such circumstances is more difficult but is more realistic. Experimental welding studies should preferably be performed on one vas of an animal while microsurgical techniques are used on the other; this allows direct comparison of the techniques in the same animal, thereby reducing the problems of biological variation.

In addition Rosemberg et al. (1985) compared his welding technique to a MSVV using only two full-thickness sutures, which may not be a fair comparison. A more realistic comparison would be between a welded technique and a MSVV using multiple sutures in either a two-layer (mucosal and sero-muscular) or "modified two-layer" (all-layer sutures plus sero-muscular layer sutures) anastomosis.

Method of Laser Tissue Welding

In this section we describe our experimental laser welding studies as an example of the technical details of the method. We have assessed the possibility of laser-assisted vasovasostomy (LAVV) bearing in mind the points raised above, and in particular attempted to answer the following questions:

1. Can laser welding of the vas be achieved reliably?
2. If so, is it also possible where there is disparity in size between the ends?
3. Are there advantages compared with a microsurgical technique in terms of:
   a) speed of procedure,
   b) reduction of sperm leakage and sperm granuloma formation,
   c) less foreign body reaction and possibly better healing,
   d) patency rates,

e) strength of the anastomosis?
4. What is the nature of the weld and how does it heal?
5. What direction should further welding research take?

Our tissue welding studies were performed using a 3-W radiofrequency excited (5-kHz) waveguide CO_2 laser, modified by the use of gallium arsenide partially reflecting mirrors to reduce the power output to between 50 and 500 mW. The laser was attached to a Leitz operating microscope (Wild M650, Heerbrugg, Switzerland). The laser was specially designed for tissue welding studies by Dr. J. Colles in the Medical Laser Unit at Herriot-Watt University, Edinburgh.

The spot size of the laser beam could be varied between 150 and 500 μm and was co-focused to the focal plane of the operating microscope. A helium–neon laser was used as an aiming beam, being aligned along the same path as the CO_2 beam so that the two beams, one invisible and one visible, could be manipulated through the operative field by the use of a joystick-controlled micromanipulator. The laser was activated by a footswitch, thus leaving both hands free for the microsurgical procedure.

Cadaver Studies

Fundamental expertise in the techniques was obtained by welding specimens of human vas obtained at post-mortem. Vasal ends were approximated in the operating field by three full-thickness sutures of 10.0 Neurilon. Using a range of spot sizes and powers the joins were assessed in terms of patency and immediate strength. Patency was tested by injecting saline and methylene blue down the lumen. Strength of the anastomosis was estimated by occluding the distal end of the vas and distending it with a mixture of water and methylene blue from a motor-driven syringe pump. A transducer was placed in line to detect pressure changes up to and after the point where the anastomosis leaked. The transducer signal drove a pen chart recorder giving a graphical representation of the intravasal pressure changes.

Animal Experimental Studies

Thirty New Zealand white rabbits underwent vasectomy under general anaesthetic. Ketamine and xylazine were administered to cause deep anaesthesia which lasted 20–30 minutes. The doses were repeated as necessary.

Twenty of the rabbits were immediately re-anastomosed (the "immediate" group) and the remaining ten underwent "delayed" reversal 8–20 weeks later when there was marked disparity in size between the two ligated ends – as is found in clinical practice. The few previous reports of experimental welding have not incorporated this important factor into the design of the study. In each animal one vas was re-anastomosed by LAVV. First three full-thickness 10.0 (0.2 metric) polyamide sutures on a 75-μm diameter round-bodied needle were used to appose the tissue edges. These sutures are convenient "guy ropes" by which to manipulate the vas without traumatising it with handling. The milliwatt CO_2 laser adapted for use with the operating microscope was set to deliver 400-mW pulses of duration 0.05 seconds and spot size 0.5 mm. These parameters produced a power density (irradiance) of 204 W/cm², an energy

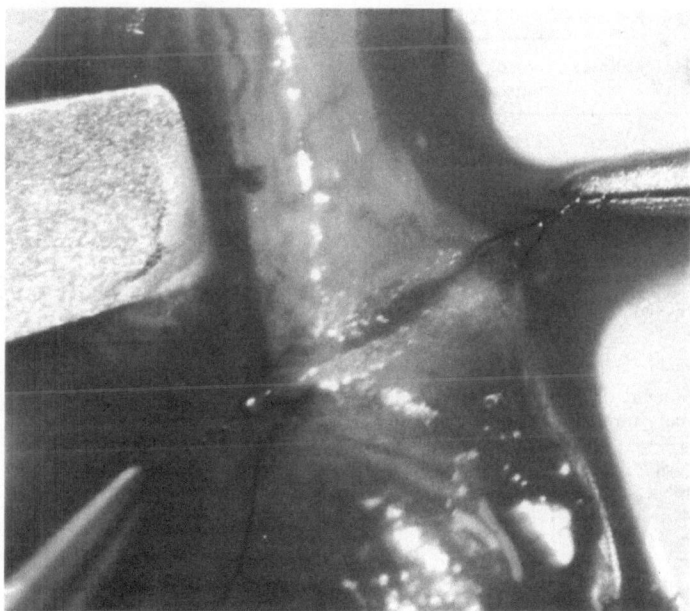

Fig. 5.12. Vasa undergoing laser welding.

density (fluence) of 10 J/cm² and a total energy of 20 mJ per pulse, and were chosen on the basis of the cadaver studies, the available literature (i.e. to achieve a power density above 40 W/cm² as shown by Rosemberg et al. (1985, 1988) for vasovasostomy and by Klink et al. (1978) for welding fallopian tubes) and the vascular welding studies undertaken in our unit (Flemming et al. 1988).

With two of the three sutures held in forceps slightly taut so as to bring the cut edges of vas together, the laser beam was focused on the apposed edges of the vas at ×40 magnification until fusion was apparent (LAVV) (Fig. 5.12). The operator sees the tissues shrink and at the same time become "sticky" so that they join across the cut edge. Laser welding continues all round the circumference of the vas, about 120–150 pulses usually being sufficient.

Contralaterally a two-layer anastomosis of 10.0 polyamide suture material (MSVV) was performed using four "all-layers" sutures placed to appose the mucosal surfaces closely, followed by five to seven sero-muscular sutures to complete the anastomosis. Times taken for the anastomosis and the number of sutures or laser pulses were recorded.

The animals were killed at 1, 4, 10 and 40 days, when patency, sperm granuloma formation and hydrostatic bursting pressures were assessed. Samples of patent anastomoses were examined by light and scanning electron microscopy.

Results

LAVV took 12 minutes compared with 19 for MSVV ($P = 0.001$) (Table 5.3). Patency rates were equally high (82.4%) for both techniques in the "immediate" group (Table 5.4) and fell to much the same extent in the technically more

Table 5.3. Treatment details for MSVV and LAVV

Technique	Anastomosis time (min)	Sutures	No. of laser pulses	Total laser energy (J)
LAVV	12 (10–20)	3	194 (120–210)	3.6 (2.4–4.2)
MSVV	19 (12–32)	9 (8–11)	NA	NA
	$P = 0.001$ (Wilcoxon signed rank test)			

Values are median and (range).
NA, not applicable.

Table 5.4. Comparative patency rates and incidence of macroscopic sperm granulomas: "immediate" reversals

Technique	Patency rate $(n = 20)$[a]	No. of sperm granulomas causing luminal narrowing
LAVV	14 (82.35%)	2
MSVV	14 (82.35%)	1

[a]Seventeen rabbits evaluable.

challenging "delayed" group (Table 5.5). Only three macroscopic sperm granulomas causing luminal narrowing were seen: two in the immediate LAVV group and one in the immediate MSVV group. Surprisingly, perhaps, none was noted in the delayed groups. Finally, bursting pressures were not significantly different whichever method of anastomosis was used (Table 5.6).

Sperm granulomas were more common in the welded anastomoses in both the study by Jarow et al. (1986) and our own, though in our experiments only marginally so and not to a statistically significant degree (2/10 in the laser group and 1/10 in the conventional). This was partly because we only counted granulomas obvious to the naked eye that were causing a stenosis at the anastomosis (McNicholas et al. 1986).

Our histological examinations showed that there was considerable damage to the tissues caused by the heat of welding, but this did not extend down to the mucosa. In our anastomoses the mucosa was often separated at the anastomotic site, but this may also be the case though less marked with a microscopic sutured technique (see Figs. 5.13 and 5.14). Others have found a similar appearance (Neblett et al. 1986; S. Thomsen, personal communication 1986). It

Table 5.5. Comparative patency rates and incidence of macroscopic sperm granulomas: "delayed" reversals

Technique	Patency rate $(n = 12)$[a]	No. of sperm granulomas causing luminal narrowing
LAVV	5 (50%)	0
MSVV	6 (60%)	0

[a]Ten rabbits evaluable.

Table 5.6. Comparative bursting pressures (mmHg): MSVV vs LAVV

Technique	Immediate[a] ($n = 10$)	Overall[b] ($n = 15$)
LAVV	72 (32–228)	78 (32–356)
MSVV	99.2 (56–254) NS[c]	99.4 (56–386) NS

[a]Immediate group only; assessed within 24 hours of anastomosis.
[b]Immediate and delayed group: assessed between 1 and 40 days after anastomosis.
[c]NS, not significant.

is not clear whether this is a phenomenon related to laser mucosal damage. As it has been reported in both welded and sutured anastomoses it may be an indication of incomplete mucosal apposition or mucosal injury at the cut edge independent of the technique used. In welded anastomoses it may be due to lack of penetration of the CO_2 laser in biological tissue so that the sutures alone will not approximate the mucosa sufficiently. One concern was that by increasing the depth of the weld we might cause delayed stricture due to more extensive scar contraction.

Discussion

A means of speeding up MSVV whilst making it easier, reducing the amount of suture material and preventing sperm leakage by creating a circumferential seal is attractive.

The variability in the techniques described and in the results of laser welding when the available literature is reviewed are not really surprising given the

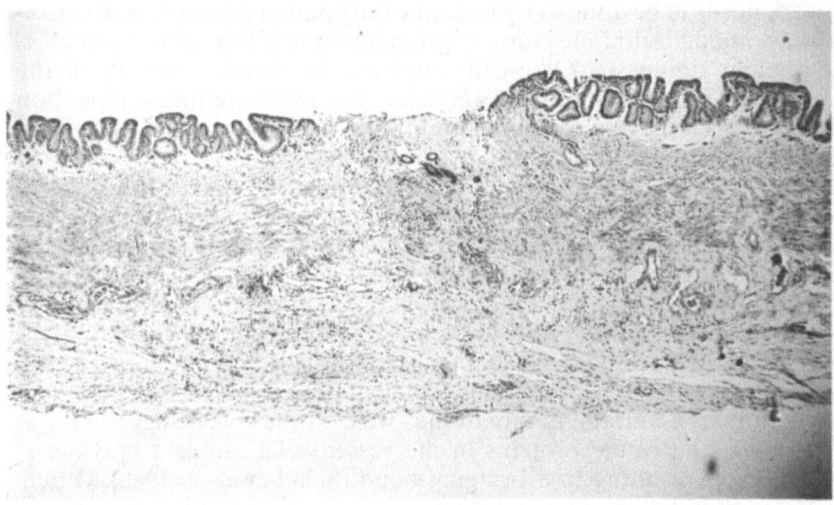

Fig. 5.13. Section through sutured anastomosis (MSVV) at 3 weeks (H&E stain).

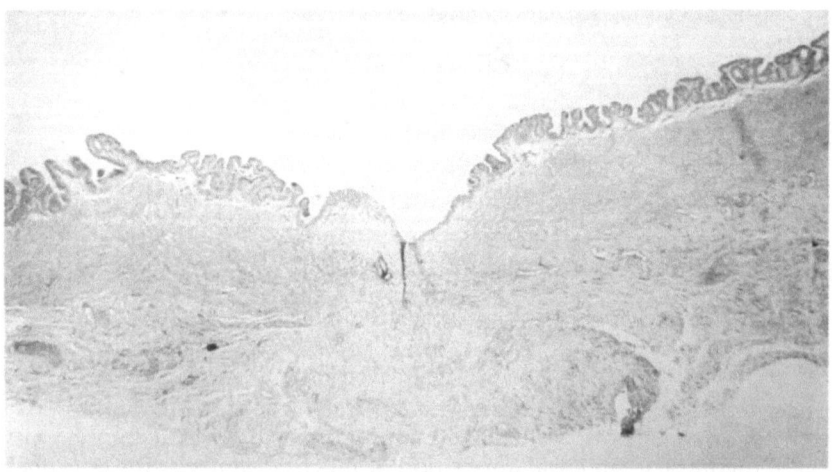

Fig. 5.14. Section through laser-welded anastomosis (LAVV) at 3 weeks (H&E stain).

large number of variables that have yet to be fully investigated. For example:

1. The reliability of the visual end point for welding, i.e. when is a weld a good weld?
2. The properties of the vessel, i.e. water content, thickness, elastic tissue content.
3. The amount of water present around the anastomotic site.
4. The position of the vessel edges relative to one another.
5. The laser parameters: fluence, irradiation time, total energy input and spot size (and, indeed, type of laser).
6. The time span between energy pulses.
7. The coaptive pressure applied to the vessel edges.

Further work needs to be done to try to define the optimal parameters for laser-assisted anastomotic techniques for any given amount of any given tissue. It is dubious whether doing so will greatly increase the tensile strength of the anastomoses, but by defining the power, spot size, exposure times, repetition rates and intervals it may be possible to minimise adjacent tissue damage and make the technique less subjective.

Since laser tissue welding is dependent on heating the tissues to the point where apposed edges stick together, the volume of tissue that requires heating is important. CO_2 laser light is strongly absorbed in water and excess water in the tissues or around them will necessitate greater energy input to raise a given volume of tissue to a given temperature. This creates problems in microsurgery as tissues are usually kept very moist. There is therefore a great deal of potentially laser-energy-absorbing water both on and adjacent to the target tissue which will complicate any attempt to calculate a precise tissue energy dose.

Debate continues about the nature of the "weld". It has been suggested that thermal denaturation of the proteins in the vessel walls causes a polymerisation of molecules resulting in a bridging bond (Schober et al. 1986). Others have suggested that the bonding is caused purely by the coagulation of blood proteins or serum proteins on the tissue surfaces forming a temporary bond and allowing repair beneath it to cause definitive joining. Indeed Almquist et al. (1984) deliberately placed a drop of blood on the outside of nerves to absorb argon laser light thereby heating tissues superficially and gluing the ends together with coagulated blood. They went on to use this method to anastomose small blood vessels in the rat (Kreuger and Almquist 1985).

The present laser technique still requires basic microsurgical skills and equipment. The laser should only be used instead of conventional techniques if there are obvious advantages in doing so. One of the major problems in vasovasostomy is the role of sperm granulomas in occlusion of the anastomosis. Since these probably occur as a result of inadequate mucosal closure it may be worth considering the use of the laser to seal the mucosal layers, reinforcing the seal with sero-muscular sutures. This would give the advantage of a watertight seal where it is most needed, with the strength of sutures to resist longitudinal forces. Alternatively the surgeon can of course accurately appose the mucosal layer with sutures. It is our finding that there is a small but significant difference in time between the two techniques which may be of value, particularly where this procedure is performed frequently.

The CO_2 laser as used in our studies is, while capable of joining two vas ends, not yet the ideal tissue welder, although further developments are likely to improve performance. The intense tissue absorption of CO_2 laser energy tended to result in superficial welding. The energy will be absorbed by any blood or water on the tissue rather than by the tissues.

A good sero-muscular weld will still not prevent sperms leaking through mucosal defects. However a wavelength with greater penetration or CO_2 lasering for longer durations at lower powers may be a better choice for creating a mucosal weld. A laser mucosal weld, if it can be achieved, may be as or more waterproof than a microsurgical mucosal anastomosis. A predominantly sero-muscular weld, as produced in this study, certainly is as waterproof as one produced with sutures.

Conclusions

1. A laser-welded anastomosis of the vas can be created using a milliwatt CO_2 laser in combination with a microsurgical technique. The weld is quicker than a sutured anastomosis, is subjectively easier and patency rates are similar. Less foreign material is left in the tissues.

2. Microsurgical skills and equipment are still necessary. The advantages in time are not overwhelming but if combined with a technically better anastomosis would be helpful to those performing this type of surgery frequently.

3. The CO_2 laser weld is predominantly located in the seromuscular layer of the vas. Thus sperms could escape through the deficient mucosal layer and cause intramural sperm granulomas.

4. Laser light of other wavelengths or the CO_2 laser used at longer pulse durations to produce a less pronounced superficial absorption and a deeper effect may prove even more useful for tissue welding of the vas.

5. Longer-term studies are needed to show details of the healing process in case circumferential scar stenosis develops.

It should not be thought that urologists are concerned solely with reversing the effects of vasectomy (or improving the fertility of rabbits and rats!) Several groups are exploring other applications of welding in urology such as CO_2 welding of the urethra (R. David, personal communication 1989), some using an egg protein as a "solder" (Poppas et al. 1988) and ureteric welding is being explored in several centres.

References

Urethral Strictures

Abdel-Hakim A, Bernstein J, Hassouna M, Elhalili MM (1983) Visual internal urethrotomy in management of urethral strictures. Urology 22:43–45

Andronaco RB, Warner RS, Cohen MS (1984) Optical urethrotomy as ambulatory procedure. Urology 24:268–270

Blandy JP (1986) Operative urology, 2nd edn. Blackwell Scientific, Oxford, pp 206–227

Bulow H (1984) Investigations of a hand held CO_2 laser connected directly to a cystoscope. Lasers Surg Med 3:308 (abstracts of the American Society for Laser Surgery and Medicine 1984)

Bulow H, Levene S (1979) Development of a CO_2 laser endoscope without a mobile arm system. Urol Res 7:31 (abstracts of 4th symposium on experimental urology 1978)

Bulow H, Bulow U, Frohmuller GW (1979a) Laser investigations of the strictured dog urethra. Invest Urol 16:403–407

Bulow H, Bulow U, Frohmuller GW (1979b) Transurethral laser urethrotomy in man: preliminary report. J Urol 121:286–287

Camey M, Le Duc A (1980) Preliminary study of the actions of the YAG laser on canine prostatic adenoma and experimental urethral stenosis. Eur Urol 6:175–179

Chilton CP, Shah PJR, Fowler CG, Tiptaft RC, Blandy JP (1983) The impact of optical urethrotomy on the management of urethral strictures. Br J Urol 55:705–710

Djulepa P, Potempa J (1983) Urethrotomy technique in urethral strictures: 6 year results. J Urol 129:955–957

Fourcade RO (1981) Endoscopic internal urethrotomy for treatment of urethral strictures. Urology 18:33

Hofstetter A, Frank F (1983) Laser use in urology. In: Dixon JA (ed) Surgical application of lasers. Year Book Medical Publishers, Chicago, ch. 8

Holm-Neilsen A, Schultz A, Moller-Pedersen V (1984) Direct vision internal urethrotomy. A critical review of 365 operations. Br J Urol 56:308–312

Matouschek E (1978) Internal urethrotomy of urethral stricture under vision. A five year report. Urol Res 6:147–150

McNicholas TA, Colles J, Bown SG, Wickham JEA (1986) CO_2 laser vaporisation of experimental urethral strictures. Presentation at the European Laser Association Meeting, Amsterdam, 6–8 Nov 1986. Laser Med Sci 1:287–288

McNicholas TA, Colles J, Bown SG, Wickham JEA (1987) CO_2 laser vaporisation of urethral strictures. Presentation at the American Urological Association annual meeting, Anaheim, USA, 17–21 May 1987. J Urol 137:176 (abstr 289)

Mundy AR, Stephenson TP (1988) Pedicled preputial patch urethroplasty. Br J Urol 61:48–51

Noske HD, Kraushaar J, Wolf M, Rothauge CF (1987) Argon laser-urethrotomy in male: results and problems. In: Waidelich W, Waidelich R (eds) Laser optoelectrics in medicine. Proceedings of the 7th congress of the International Society for Laser Surgery and Medicine, Munich 1987. Springer, Berlin Heidelberg New York, pp 327–328

Perez-Castro EE, Martinez-Pinero JA (1982) Endoscopic urethrotomy plus laser photocoagulation in urethral strictures. Read at 19th international conference of the Société Internationale d'Urologie, San Francisco, abstr 473

Ravasini G (1957) Die kontrollierte urethroskopische Elektrotomie für die Behandlung von Harnrohrenstrikturen. Urologia 24:229–231

Rogers HS, McNicholas TA, Fowler CG, Blandy JP (1988) Long term results of 203 one stage island patch urethroplasties. Presentation at the European Association of Urology. London. 18–21 May 1988 (abstr 296)

Rothauge C (1980) Urethroscopic recanalisation of urethral stenosis using argon laser. Urology 16:158–161

Sachse HE (1974) Zur Behandlung der Harnrohrenstriktur: die transurethrale Schlitzung unter Sicht mit scharfen Schnitt. Fortschr Med 92:12–15

Sacknoff EJ (1985) CO_2 laser cystoscopy. Lasers Surg Med 5:162 (abstr)

Shanberg AM, Chalfin SA, Tansey LA (1984) Nd-YAG laser: new treatment for urethral stricture disease. Urology 24:15

Shanberg A, Baghdassarian R, Tansey L, Sawyer D (1988) KTP laser in treatment of urethral strictures. Urology 32:517–520

Shulman D, Aronson HB (1984) Capnography in the early diagnosis of carbon dioxide embolism during laparoscopy. Can Anaesth Soc J 31:455–459

Singh M, Blandy JP (1976) The pathology of urethral stricture. J Urol 115:673–676

Smith JA, Dixon JA (1984) Nd-YAG laser treatment of benign urethral strictures. J Urol 131:1080–1081

Smith PJB, Roberts JBM, Ball AJ, Kaisary AV (1983) Long term results of optical urethrotomy. Br J Urol 55:698–700

Smith PJB, Kaisary AV, Ball AJ (1984) Late results of optical urethrotomy. J R Soc Med 77:105–107

Turner-Warwick RT (1987) Urethral stricture surgery. In: Mundy AR (ed) Current operative surgery: urology. Ballière Tindall, Eastbourne

Turner-Warwick RT (1988) A critical review of the principles of urethrotomy: its complications and their surgical resolution. Presentation at the EAU London. 18–21 May 1988 (abstr 295)

Wilscher MK (1985) Endoscopic delivery of laser energy. In: Smith JA (ed) Lasers in urologic surgery. Year Book Publishers, Chicago, pp 143–149

Wilscher MK, Filso AM, Jako GJ, Olsson CA (1978) Development of a carbon dioxide laser cystoscope. J Urol 119:202–207

Zincke H, Furlow WL (1985) Long term results in transpubic urethroplasty. J Urol 133:605

Condylomatous Disease

Baggish MS (1985) Improved laser techniques for the elimination of genital and extragenital warts. Am J Obstet Gynecol 153:545–550

Campion MJ, Clarkson PK, Singer A, McCance DJ (1985) Increased risk of cervical neoplasia in consorts of men with penal condylomata acuminata. Lancet i:943–946

Crum CP, Egawa K, Barron B et al. (1983) Human papilloma virus infection (condyloma) of the cervix and cervical intraepithelial neoplasia: a histological and statistical analysis. Gynecol Oncol 15:88–97

Haddad NG, Hussein IY, Livingstone JRB, Smart GE (1988) Colposcopy in teenagers. Br Med J 297:29–30

Lundquist SG, Lindstedt EM (1983) Laser treatment of condylomata acuminata. Lasers Surg Med 3:152–154 (abstr)

Meandzija MP (1985) The technique of carbon dioxide laser management of condyloma acuminatum. Lasers Med Chir 1:5–12

Riva JM, Sedlacek TV, Cunnane MF, Mangan CE (1989) Extended carbon dioxide laser vaporisation in the treatment of subclinical papillomavirus infection of the lower genital tract. Obstet Gynecol 73:25–30

Rosemberg SK (1985) Carbon dioxide laser treatment of external genital lesions. Urology 25:555–558

Urethral Haemangiomas

Amagai T, Onoe Y, Okada K (1981) Laser application for urological disease. Presentation to the 4th International Congress of Laser Medicine and Surgery, Tokyo 1981

Miller RA, Coptcoat MJ, Parry J, Dawkins G, Wickham JEA (1987) The integrated cystoscope: an alternative to conventional and fibreoptic cystoscopy. Br J Urol 60:128–131

Senoh K, Miyazaki T, Kikuchi I, Sumiyoshy A, Kohga A (1981) Haemangiomatous lesions of the glans penis. Urology 17:194–196

Smith JA, Dixon JA (1984) Laser treatment of bladder haemangioma. Urology 24:134
Tilak GH (1967) Multiple haemangioma of the male urethra: treatment by Denis Browne-Swinney-Johanson urethroplasty. J Urol 97:96–97

Tissue Anastomosis and Repair

Almquist EE, Nathemson A, Auth D, Almquist B, Hall S (1984) Evaluation of the use of the argon laser in repairing rat and primate nerves. J Hand Surg 9:792–799
Androsov PI (1956) New method of surgical treatment of blood vessel lesions. Arch Surg 73:902–910
Belker AM (1985) The use of carbon dioxide laser in microsurgery. Urology 25:432 (letter)
Blakemore AH, Stefko PL, Lord JW Jr (1942) The severed primary artery in the war wounded. A non-suture method of blood vessel anastomosis. Surgery 12:488–508
Blakemore AH, Stefko PL, Lord JW Jr (1943) Restoration of blood flow in damaged arteries: further studies on a non-suture method of blood vessel anastomosis. Ann Surg 117:481–497
Carter EL, Roth EJ (1958) Direct non-suture method of small vein anastomoses in the dog. Ann Surg 148:212–218
Cobett JR (1967) Microvascular surgery. Surg Clin N Am 47:521–542
Cos LR, Valvo JR, Davis RS, Cockett ATK (1983) Vasovasostomy: current state of the art. Urology 22:567–575
Derrick FC, Yarbrough W, D'Agostino J (1973) Vasovasostomy: results of questionnaire of members of the American urological association. J Urol 110:556–557
Dew DK (1983) Nd-YAG and CO_2 laser closure of rat skin incisions. Lasers Surg Med 3:109
Dew DK (1984) Laser microsurgical repair of soft tissues: a demonstration of surgical techniques. Lasers Surg Med 3:351 (abstr 140)
Dew DK (1986) Review and status report on laser tissue fusion. SPIE Lasers Med 712:255–257
Dew DK, Serbent RH, Art WS, Boynton GC, Byrne JD, Evans TA, Hirshberg JG, Wouters AW, Hernandes A (1983) Laser assisted microsurgical vessel anastomosis techniques: the use of the argon and CO_2 lasers. Lasers Med Surg 3:132 and 145 (abstr)
Fisher SE, Frame JW, Bronwe RM, Tranter RMD (1983) A comparative histological study of wound healing following CO_2 laser conventional surgical excision of canine buccal mucosal wounds. Arch Oral Biol 28:287–291
Flemming AFS, Colles MJ, Guillanotti R (1988) Laser assisted microvascular anastomosis of arteries and veins: laser tissue welding. Br J Plast Surg 41:378–388
Goetz RH, Lissberg R, Hoppenstein R (1966) Vascular necrosis caused by application of methyl-2-cyanoacrylate (Eastman 1910 monomer). Ann Surg 63:243–248
Hagan KF, Coffey DS (1977) The adverse effects of sperm during vasovasostomy. J Urol 118:269–271
Hagstrom H, Hagland H (1985) Post-operative decrease in suture holding capacity in laparotomy wounds and anastomoses. Act Chir Scand 151:533–535
Hopfner E (1903) Über Gefaessnacht, Gefaesstransplantation und Reimplantation von amputierten Extremitaeten. Arch Klin Chir 70:417–454
Hosbein DJ, Blumenstock DH (1964) Anastomoses of small arteries using tissue adhesives. Surg Gynecol Obstet 118:112–114
Huang C, Chow SPM, Chan CW (1982) Experience with anastomoses of arteries approximately 0.02 mm in external diameter. Plast Reconstr Surg 69:299–305
Inokuchi K (1961) Stapling device for end-to-side anastomosis of blood vessels. Arch Surg 82:337–342
Jacobsen JH, Surez EL (1960) Microsurgery of anastomoses of small vessels. Surg Forum 11:243–245
Jain KK (1983) Sutureless end-to-side microvascular anastomosis using Nd:YAG laser. Vasc Surg 17:240–243
Jain KK, Gorish W (1979) Repair of small blood vessels with the Nd:YAG laser: a preliminary report. Surgery 85:684–688
Jarrow JP, Cooley BC, Marshall FF (1986) Laser assisted vasal anastomoses in the rat and man. J Urol 36:1132–1135
Karl P, Tilgner A, Heiner H (1981) A new adhesive technique for microvascular anastomoses: a preliminary report. Br J Plast Surg 34:61–63
Klink F, Grosspietzsch R, von Klitzing L, Endell W, Husstedt W, Oberheuser F (1978) Animal in vivo and in vitro experiments with human tube ends for end to end anastomotic operation by CO_2 laser technique. Fertil Steril 30:100–102

Kreuger RR, Almquist EE (1985) Argon laser coagulation of blood for the anastomosis of small blood vessels. Lasers Surg Med 5:55–60

Kuss R, Gregoire W (1988) Histoire illustrée de l'urologie. Editions Roger Costa, Paris

Lexer E (1907) Die ideale Operation des arteriallen und des arteriellvenosen Aneurysma. Arch Klin Chir 83:459–477

Lidman D, Daniel RK (1981) Evaluation of clinical microvascular anastomoses: reasons for failure. Ann Plast Surg 6:215–223

Luke M, Kvist E, Andersen F, Hjortrup A (1986) Reduction of postoperative bleeding after TUR by local instillation of fibrin adhesive (Beriplast). Br J Urol 58:672–675

Lynne CM, Carter M, Morris J, Dew DK, Thomsen S, Thomsen C (1983) Laser assisted vas anastomoses: a preliminary report. Lasers Surg Med 3:261–263

McNicholas TA, Flemming AFS, Cross FW, Colles JC, Bown SG, Wickham JEA, Clark CG (1986) Laser assisted vasovasostomy (LAVV): an experimental study. Presentation to the 21st Congress of the European Society for Surgical Research, Nancy, France, 6–9 May 1986. Eur Surg Res 18 [Suppl 1]:84–85

McNicholas TA, Flemming S, Colles J, Cross FW, Bown SG (1987) Laser assisted vasovasostomy. Presentation to the American Urological Association annual meeting, Anaheim, USA, 17–21 May 1987. J Urol 137:163 (abstr 238)

Murphy LJT (1972) The history of urology. CC Thomas, Springfield, Illinois

Nakayama K, Yamamoto K, Makino H (1963) A new vascular anastomosis instrument: a clinical approach. Clin Orthop 29:123–131

Neblett CR, Morris JR, Thomsen S (1986) Laser assisted microsurgical anastomosis. Neurosurgery 19:914–934

O'Conor V (1948) Anastomosis of the vas deferens after purposeful division for sterility. J Urol 59:229–231

Payr E (1900) Beiträge zur Technik der Blutgefass und Nervennaht nebst Mitteilungen über die Verwendung eines resorbirbaren Metalles in der Chirurgie. Arch Klin Chir 62:67–93

Poppas DP, Schlossberg SM, Richmond IL, Gilbert DA, Devine CJ (1988) Laser welding in urethral surgery: improved results with a protein solder. J Urol 139:415–417

Proust R (1904) La prostatectomie dans l'hypertrophie de la prostate. Naud, Paris

Que MY, Sigel B (1965) Electrocoaptive closure of linear incision in veins. Surgery 58:679–681

Quigley MR, Bailes JE, Kwaan HC, Cerullo LJ (1985) Laser assisted vascular anastomosis. Lancet i:334

Rosemberg SK (1987) Clinical use of carbon dioxide (CO_2) laser in microsurgical vasovasostomy. Urology 29:372–374

Rosemberg SK, Elson L, Lawrence EN (1985) Carbon dioxide laser microsurgical vasovasostomy. Urology 25:53–56

Rosemberg SK, Elson LM, Nathan EL (1988) Laser vasovasostomy. A comparative retrospective study using Bioquantum microsurgical carbon dioxide laser. Urology 31:237–239

Schober R, Ulrich F, Sander T, Durselen H, Hessel S (1986) Laser induced alteration of collagen substructure allows microsurgical tissue welding. Science 232:1421–1422

Sharlip ID (1981) Vasovasostomy: comparison of two microsurgical techniques. Urology 17:347–352

Silber SJ (1984) Microsurgery for vasectomy reversal and vasoepididymostomy. Urology 23:505–528

Stein BS, Cooley BC (1988) Carbon dioxide laser assisted microscopic vasovasostomy. J Endourology 2:299–307

Sushruta samihita, 600 BC (1969) The classic reprint: Ancient ear-lobe and rhinoplastic operations in India. Plast Reconstr Surg 43:515–522

Yahr WZ, Strully KJ (1967) Effects of laser on blood vessel wall. A method of non-occlusive vascular anastomosis. In: Donaghy RMP, Yasargil MG (eds) Microvascular surgery. CV Mosby, St Louis/Georg Thieme Verlag, Stuttgart, pp 135–137

Chapter 6

Photodynamic Therapy

R. O. Plail, J. I. Harty and H. B. Lottmann

Introduction

Photodynamic therapy (PDT) is an experimental form of cancer treatment which has been used to treat a variety of human cancers including transitional cell carcinoma of the bladder (Dougherty 1986). A simplified scheme of the principles of PDT is shown in Fig. 6.1.

A patient with tumour is injected intravenously with a photosensitising drug which circulates throughout the body, including tumour tissue. After an appropriate interval, the tumour is illuminated with laser light at a wavelength which coincides with the excitation wavelength of the sensitiser (the wavelength at which the photosensitiser is activated). The light energy is taken up by the sensitiser and, by a photochemical reaction in the presence of oxygen, cell destruction occurs. There may be damage to surrounding normal tissue which is also sensitised and skin sensitivity may remain for some time.

Tumour damage in PDT has variously been attributed to selective uptake (Gomer and Dougherty 1979) or selective retention of sensitiser (Jocham et al. 1984), or to relatively similar damage to both neoplastic and normal tissue but with recovery of the normal tissue. There is evidence that both direct cellular effects (Dougherty 1984) and vascular damage (Selman et al. 1985) occur. Both singlet oxygen (Weishaupt et al. 1976), a toxic oxygen radical, and free radicals (Foote 1984), formed by electron transfer reactions between excited states of the photosensitiser and cellular substrates, may be responsible for the photodynamic effect. However, at present the exact mechanism of tumour destruction is not well defined.

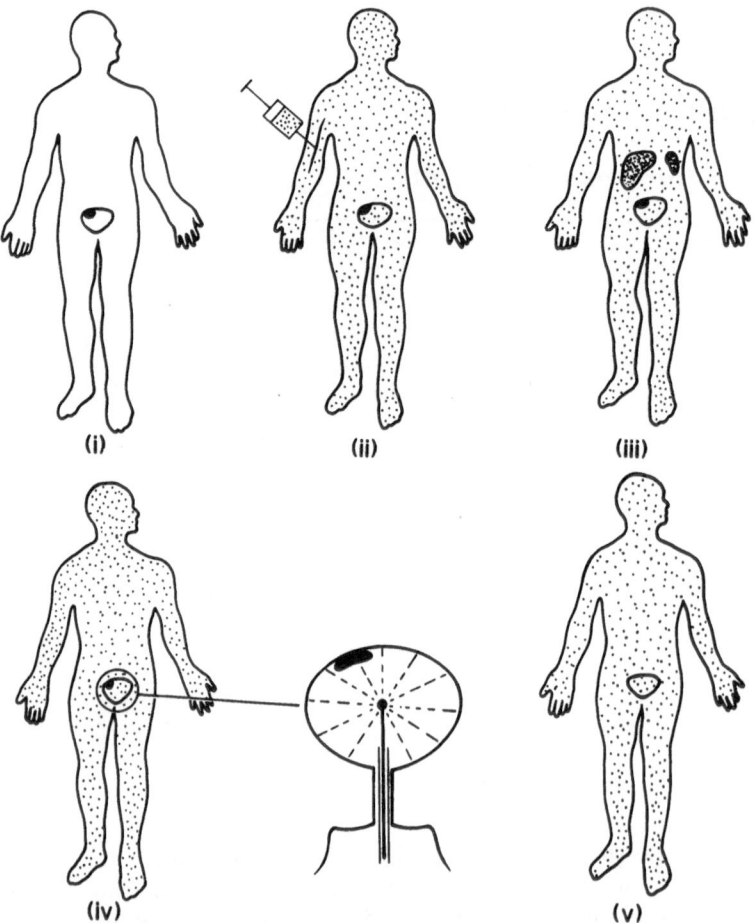

Fig. 6.1. Simplified scheme of the principles for PDT in superficial bladder cancer.

Historical Background

The ability of photosensitisers to cause a photochemical reaction has been recognised since the beginning of the twentieth century. In 1900, Raab used acridine orange and eosin to destroy *Paramecium* on exposure to light. In 1903, Tappeiner and Jesionek treated skin tumours following topical application of eosin and exposure to white light. Policard (1924) noted that certain tumours contained intrinsic porphyrins which, when exposed to ultraviolet light, produced a red fluorescence. In 1942, Auler and Banzer reported selective fluorescence in implanted rat tumours following systemically administered haematoporphyrin (Hp) and ultraviolet illumination. However, the evidence for their claims of increased tumour necrosis and reduced tumour mass compared with controls was inconclusive.

Haematoporphyrin was shown to be a crude mixture of porphyrins and the localising elements were the "impurities" in the mixture rather than the Hp (Lipson et al. 1961). Lipson and colleagues therefore used haematoporphyrin derivative (HpD) in order to eliminate the effects of using the crude mixture. HpD, made by treating Hp with sulphuric acid and acetic acid, was shown to have an enhanced affinity for malignant cells and to localise in several different human tumours. Later, Lipson et al. (1967) reported successfully treating a human breast cancer using a xenon lamp after systemic administration of HpD.

Dougherty et al. (1975) caused damage in mouse mammary tumours using HpD and red light from a xenon arc lamp. Kelly and Snell (1976) were the first to show the therapeutic potential of PDT in bladder cancer. They treated a patient with superficial bladder cancer with HpD and red light from a mercury lamp, by transmitting the light into the bladder through a glass light-guide within a cystoscope sheath. Destruction of tumours was seen at cystoscopy several days later.

In the UK, approximately 10 000 new patients per year present with transitional cell carcinoma of the bladder (OPCS 1988), of whom 50%–60% develop recurrent superficial disease (Heney et al. 1982). Repeated resection and fulguration in conjunction with intravesical chemotherapy is initially effective in controlling tumours in approximately 66% of patients in the first year, but this percentage later diminishes (Glashan 1987).

It is appropriate, therefore, to investigate the possible role of other methods of treatment such as PDT. With existing photosensitisers and light delivery systems, a photodynamic effect can be produced in the bladder and it thus has therapeutic potential.

Photosensitisers

HpD has been most widely used both clinically and experimentally, but it is a complex, unstable mixture of different porphyrins (Bonnett et al. 1981). These are based on a tetrapyrrole ring to which are added various side chains (Fig. 6.2). The nature of the active component of HpD is disputed (Berenbaum et al. 1982; Kessel 1986). Dougherty has championed the claims of a partially purified material, thought to contain a higher percentage of the active ingredients of HpD, which are supposed to be dihaematoporphyrin ether or ester (DHE) (Dougherty et al. 1984).

The phthalocyanines comprise a second group of sensitisers which have been used extensively experimentally but not in clinical practice (Ben-Hur and Rosenthal 1985; Bown et al. 1986). These agents are porphyrin-like synthetic dyes. The metallophthalocyanines, especially the aluminium and zinc derivatives, have electron configurations which make them efficient sensitisers. With maximal absorption at longer light wavelengths (e.g. 675 nm), deeper tissue penetration may be achieved. Their major importance may lie in the apparently low risk of cutaneous photosensitivity associated with their use and the possibility that they exert a "collagen sparing" effect, at least in the rodent gut (Barr et al. 1987a, b).

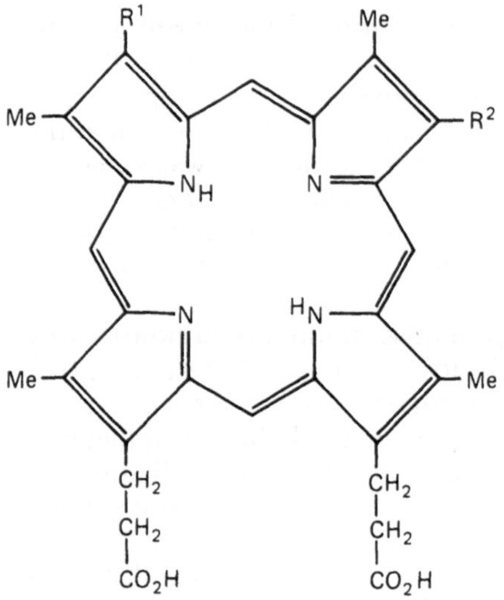

Fig. 6.2. The porphyrin tetrapyrrole ring to which are added subgroups (R^1 and R^2) to form the components of HpD.

Selectivity of Uptake

The complex nature of HpD and the uncertainty about the nature of the active fraction make assays difficult. The main methods used to measure HpD concentrations are fluorescence detection and autoradiographic techniques. Fluorescence studies are performed by illuminating the sensitised tissues, usually with ultraviolet light, and detecting the longer wavelength fluorescent light which is emitted (Lin et al. 1984). Autoradiography involves tagging HpD with a radioactive label (Gomer and Dougherty 1979). There is some evidence of increased fluorescence corresponding to areas of malignancy (Gregorie et al. 1968) but some frankly malignant areas in the bladder show no fluorescence whereas oedematous, traumatised or regenerating tissues often show the strongest fluorescence (Kelly and Snell 1976; Selman et al. 1985).

In mouse tissues and in a transplanted mammary carcinoma, Gomer and Dougherty (1979) detected radiolabelled HpD in (in order of decreasing concentration) liver, spleen, tumour, skin and muscle. Liver and spleen do not fluoresce with any intensity, largely due to their pigmentation which quenches the fluorescence. Thus, fluorescence detection may delineate areas of tumour but it is an unreliable indicator of HpD concentration. In addition, the active fraction of HpD is not known and there is no certainty that increased concentrations of HpD equate with photosensitiser activity.

The evidence for selective tumour uptake of HpD is therefore weak. There may be selective retention of HpD by tumours (Jocham et al. 1984a) but this evidence is based on spectrofluorimetric data which is unreliable for a mixture such as HpD due to the same limitations described above. In fact it may be that the most reliable assay for the active element of HpD is its biological effect in vivo.

Selectivity of Effect

Kelly et al. (1975), using human bladder tumour cells and normal transitional cells implanted subcutaneously in immunosuppressed mice, showed that HpD and white light from an iodide lamp destroyed the tumours but not normal tissue.

Jocham et al. (1984a) performed intravesical PDT on Brown-Pearce carcinomas implanted submucosally in rabbit bladders and found destruction of 19 of 22 tumours with no adverse effects on the normal urothelium. However, these tumours are known to regress spontaneously and no control animals were used. The same workers (Jocham et al. 1984b) found no damage to normal rat bladders illuminated 24–60 hours after sensitisation with HpD, whereas they reported complete destruction of 13 out of 14 BBN-induced rat bladder tumours treated at the same interval. The experimental details are, however, unclear. Contrary to the above findings, Plail et al. (1988), using an MNU-induced rat bladder tumour model (Severs et al. 1982), showed that there was little tumour selectivity. Tumours were treated with HpD 20 mg/kg 24–72 hours before illumination with light at 511 and 578 nm at power densities of 200 mW/cm^2 and light doses of 10–80 J/cm^2. The tumours were damaged, with up to 2 mm depth of necrosis (Figs. 6.3 and 6.4), but the normal bladder was also damaged. However, despite sustaining full-thickness necrosis, the normal rat bladder wall recovered after several weeks with complete restitution and no scarring.

There are, to date, no other comparable animal studies. These results and the clinical results discussed below, suggest that there is little selective tumoricidal effect in the bladder. However, papillary tumours can be at least partially damaged. The damage caused to the rest of the bladder may be beneficial in treating areas of carcinoma in situ or areas of unstable urothelium.

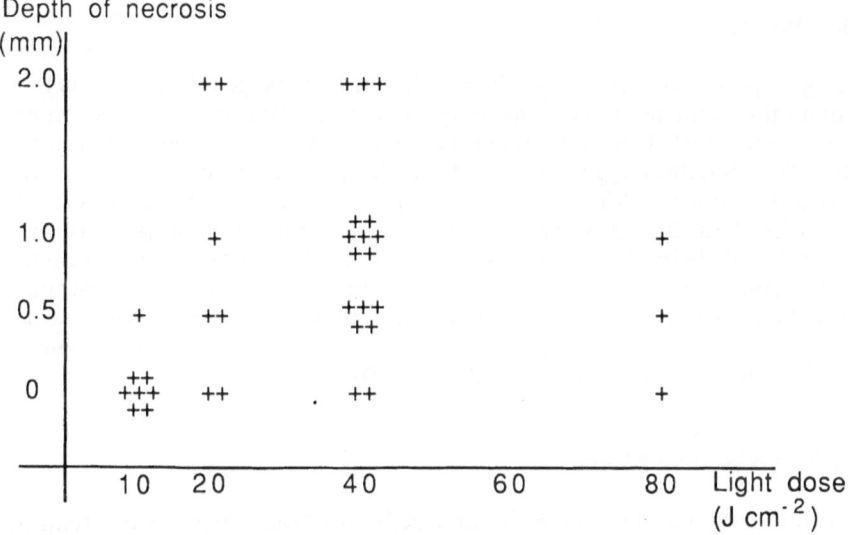

Fig. 6.3. The effect of light dose on tumour necrosis. (MNU-induced rat bladder tumours, HpD sensitised 24–72 hours before illumination at 511/578 nm, 200 mW/cm^2. Animals were killed 24 hours after illumination.)

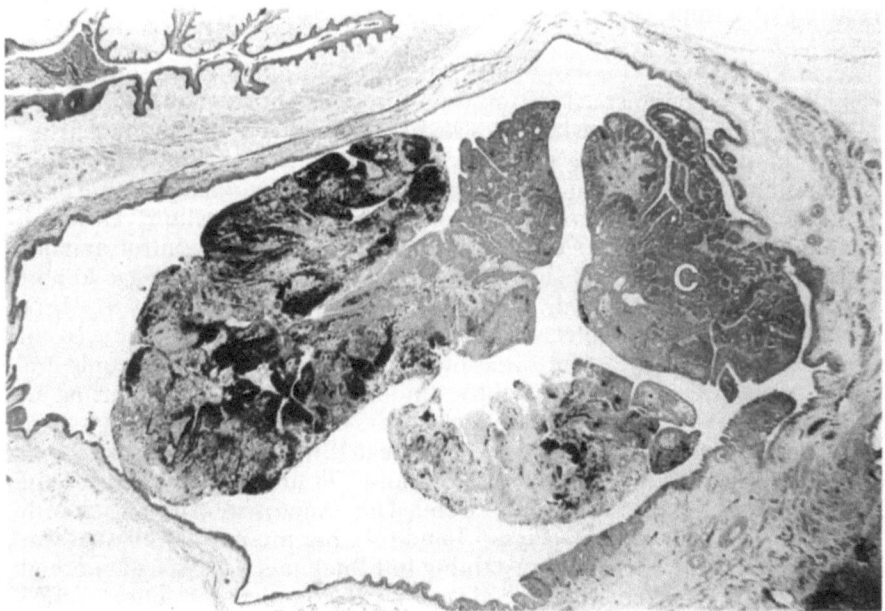

Fig. 6.4. Necrosis of rat bladder tumour after PDT compared with adjacent non-illuminated control tumour (*C*). (HpD 20 mg/kg 24 hours before illumination at 511/578 nm, 200 mW/cm², 40 J/cm². H&E, ×5.)

Mechanism of Action of PDT

Tissue Oxygen

Several groups of workers have shown that tissue oxygen is necessary for photodynamic damage to occur, as temporary ischaemia of the treated organ or tumour during PDT eliminates cell damage (Bown et al. 1986; Gomer and Razum 1984). Singlet oxygen, a toxic radical, appears to be involved in the photodynamic process although the evidence is largely circumstantial as it is a very short-lived entity and is present in minute amounts for short periods only (Weishaupt et al. 1976). Free radicals (Foote 1984), formed by electron transfer reactions between excited states of the photosensitiser and cellular substrates, may also be partly responsible for the photodynamic effect. What does seem clear is that peroxidation of polyunsaturated fatty acids occurs with consequent disruption of cell membranes (Spikes 1984).

Direct Non-vascular Effect

Several authors have demonstrated that cells are killed in vitro by treating them with HpD and light of appropriate wavelength, which suggests a direct cytotoxic effect of PDT (Diamond et al. 1972; Gomer and Smith 1980). There are reports of damage to cell membranes (Malik and Djaldetti 1980; Bellnier and Dougherty 1982). Other cell components have been shown to be damaged including mitochondria, endoplasmic reticulum and the nuclear membrane (Moan 1986). Berenbaum et al. (1986b) described the effect of PDT on the endothelial cells of small vessels as causing cell separation and increased vesiculation of the endothelium. This endothelial damage is thought to contribute to vascular damage in sensitised tissues.

Direct Vascular Effect

Henderson et al. (1984) demonstrated a possible direct vascular effect by examining the survival of tumour cells at increasing intervals following treatment with HpD and light in vivo. There was no reduction in survival of cells cultured from the tumour immediately after treatment. However, the survival of cells taken from tumours several hours after treatment fell substantially, suggesting an ischaemic effect of PDT. This was paralleled by killing animals and taking tumour cells at intervals post-mortem. Selman et al. (1984) studied the effects of HpD and light on blood flow in transplantable FANFT-induced urothelial tumours in the rat bladder. They found that treatment caused a significant decrease in tumour blood flow and in a later study (Selman et al. 1985) showed a positive correlation between reduction in tumour blood flow and tumour regression. Bugelski et al. (1981) found that red blood cells escaped through damaged vessel walls in experimental animal tumours within 15 minutes of PDT. Using "sandwich" observation chambers, Star et al. (1984) studied the effects of PDT on the microcirculation in RMA-rat mammary carcinomas and demonstrated destruction of normal and tumour vessels that they concluded contributed to tumour kill. Thus, small vessel damage and subsequent reduction in blood supply appear to be important factors in the cytotoxic effect of PDT.

Thermal or Photodynamic Effect?

The histological effects of PDT are similar to those caused by hyperthermia but PDT damage occurs at lower light doses and power densities. Svaasand (1985) found both thermal and photodynamic damage in experimental models, the relative contributions being dependent on the depth of tissue treated and partly on the light dosimetry. Hyperthermic damage was more evident at higher power densities. In our own laboratories, we found thermal damage in normal unsensitised rat bladders treated with light at 511/578 nm at power densities of approximately 400 mW/cm² and a light dose of 80 J/cm², whereas after sensitisation a photodynamic effect was observed at 200 mW/cm² and 10 J/cm² (Plail et al. 1988).

Treatment Parameters

Light Wavelength

The wavelength of the light source in PDT is chosen to coincide with the excitation wavelengths of the sensitiser. Many workers have preferred red light (625–630 nm) as it activates HpD, albeit at a weak excitation peak, and it penetrates tissue to a depth of several millimetres. In 1985, van Gemert et al. described the relative depths of necrosis in transplanted mouse tumours treated with HpD and light at three wavelengths: 405 nm (the Soret band), 514.5 nm (green) and 630 nm (red). They confirmed the greater penetration of red light but found that at depths of 2–3 mm or less, green light was more efficient in destroying tumours. The less penetrating green light would appear to be ideally suited to the treatment of superficial bladder tumours.

Optimal Timing of Treatment

Gomer and Dougherty (1979) showed that maximum porphyrin levels in all tissues analysed were obtained within 3–4 hours, followed by stable concentrations for the next 44–45 hours. Lottmann et al. (1988) found maximum concentrations of aluminium sulphonated phthalocyanine (AlSPC) in rat bladder muscle and mucosa at 3–48 hours after injection of AlSPC 5 mg/kg, and they also found significant concentrations up to 15 days later. It appears from this and other data that the interval from sensitisation to treatment may not be critical. Most clinical studies have been performed 24–72 hours after sensitisation.

Light Dosage

Nseyo et al. (1985) studied the effects of PDT on the normal canine bladder. They found that power densities of approximately 400 mW/cm^2 and a light dose of 18–30 J/cm^2 caused a photodynamic effect in the submucosa and mucosa with only minimal damage to the muscle. Plail et al. (1988), as discussed above, showed that a power density of 200 mW/cm^2 and a light dose of 20–40 J/cm^2 caused tumour necrosis up to a depth of 2 mm in rat bladder tumours, 24 hours after sensitisation with HpD (Fig. 6.3). Lottmann et al. (1988) found a marked reduction in rat bladder capacity after administration of AlSPC 2.5 mg/kg followed by whole bladder illumination at 671 nm, light doses of 25–100 J/cm^2 and power densities of 80 mW/cm^2, delivered 3–72 hours after sensitisation. This contraction resulted in vesicoureteral reflux, hydroureteronephrosis, renal abscesses (Fig. 6.5) and death of the rats within 7 days. Histology of the bladder showed full-thickness necrosis except for the collagen in the submucosa which was relatively spared. Cystometrographic studies showed a loss of bladder compliance with raised intravesical pressure leading to vesicoureteral reflux (Fig. 6.6).

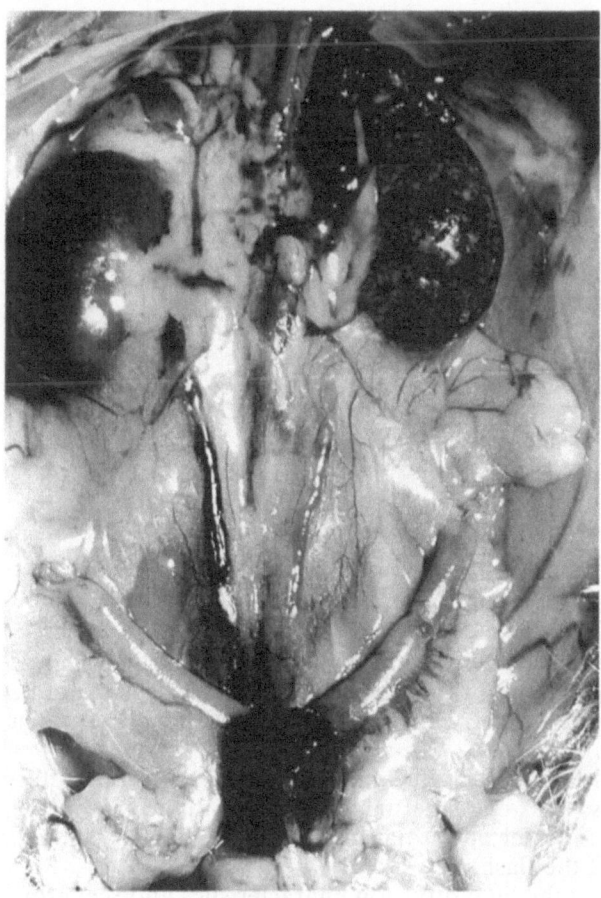

Fig. 6.5. Hydroureteronephrosis and renal abscesses in a rat given PDT. (AlSPC 2.5 mg/kg 24 hours before illumination at 671 nm, 80 mW/cm^2, 25 J/cm^2.)

Light Distribution

We have attempted to determine the optimum treatment parameters in animal models, and have each found that the normal animal bladder is susceptible to damage. This makes for difficult light dosimetry control in treating patients, and a major part of our work has been the investigation of light distribution in bladder models. Hollow organs, such as the urinary bladder, pose special problems in delivering an optimum light isodose distribution to all areas of the mucosa. The dose is critical to ensure that tumours are destroyed but that the normal bladder urothelium is spared, and as the bladder is rarely spherical, the dose is difficult to control. Several solutions to the problem have been investigated.

Hisazumi et al. (1984) designed an elaborate system comprising an optical fibre which delivered light onto a conical mirror mounted at the end of a cystoscope. The light was delivered onto the bladder mucosa in sections and by

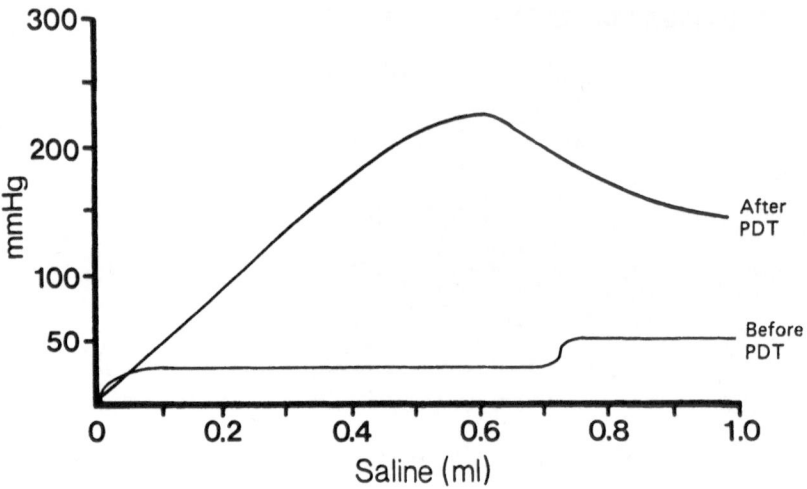

Fig. 6.6. Rat bladder capacity and intravesical pressure before and after PDT.

withdrawing the device at a calculated rate, the whole bladder urothelium was illuminated. However, some regions of the fundus and bladder base might be left untreated and the bladder geometry might result in considerable errors in dosage.

Jocham et al. (1984a) and Baghdassarian et al. (1985) achieved uniform illumination in a spherical glass flask by scattering light using a dilute suspension of Intralipid (Kabivitrum) in water and a flat-tipped optical fibre positioned with the tip in the centre of the flask.

Lottmann (1987) compared the light diffusion characteristics and scattering efficiency of a square-ended optical fibre in Intralipid alone and a bulb-tipped fibre which comprised a 5.5-mm diameter glass bulb containing 10% Intralipid. He used either a white-clad or a black-clad flask and measured the space irradiance at the surface through small windows cut in the cladding. Measurements were made for each tip in each of the two flasks and the results recorded on polar plots using an arbitrary power density unit.

As reported by others, Lottmann concluded that the position of the light source was critical in achieving an isotropic light distribution and that of the two tips, the bulb tip was more efficient in respect of total light dose delivered at the surface of the flask. The optimum position for the bare fibre tip in Intralipid was found to be one-quarter of the distance from the centre to the neck of the flask; the optimum position of the second system was at the centre of the flask (Fig. 6.7). A 1-cm alteration of tip position resulted in complete loss of uniform light distribution at the flask surface.

Lottmann found that the light distribution within the white flask was slightly more isotropic than in the black flask, suggesting that internal reflection at the bladder surface improved the homogeneity of irradiation. Isodose illumination at the flask neck was difficult to achieve, suggesting the need for a separate light source application at the bladder neck.

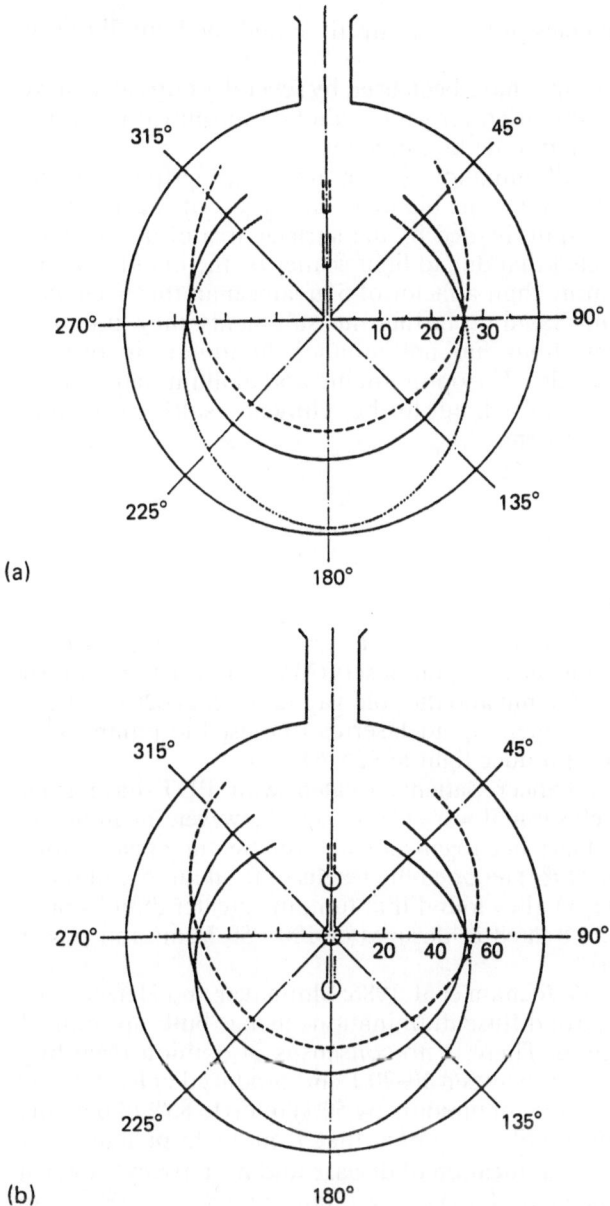

Fig. 6.7. Polar plots of a baré fibre (a) and a bulb-tip fibre (b) in a spherical flask showing the optimum tip position and the effect of a 1-cm change in position.

By measuring the total energy transmission at the surface of the black-clad flask, the bulb-tip fibre was found to be 4 times more efficient than the bare fibre, indicating a greater light transmission efficiency for the bulb-tip design. In the white-clad flask, the total light transmission of both systems was markedly increased, presumably due to internal reflection from the white surface. The ratio of the efficiencies of the bulb-tip fibre and the bare fibre was 2 : 1.

Composite diffusing "bulb-tips" have been used by several groups to achieve uniform scatter, but the maximum power which can be transmitted is limited by the nature of the materials and the bonding agent.

With intracavitary bladder illumination and optimum scattering, it is customary to determine the light dose at the bladder wall by a simple calculation of the primary light beam output divided by the surface area of the bladder. Star et al. (1987) have suggested that due to light scatter by the bladder tissue, the true light dose may be more than a factor of 5 greater than the calculated dose from the primary beam. Based on further measurements, they have also suggested that the use of Intralipid may not enhance the uniformity of light scatter within an irregular bladder. The optimum method of illumination in an irregular bladder remains unresolved, but further clinical results will help to determine the most effective system.

Clinical Studies

Previous clinical studies have utilised two laser systems: the argon-ion laser emitting light at 534 nm and the metal vapour lasers (MVL) of which the copper vapour laser emits at 511 and 578 nm and the gold vapour laser at 628 nm. Both the argon-ion laser and the copper vapour laser can be used to pump a dye laser and, with suitable dyes, produce light at 625–635 nm.

Several series of bladder cancer patients treated with PDT have been reported since Kelly and Snell's initial work (Table 6.1). However, the numbers are small, the pathological stages heterogeneous and the treatment conditions very variable. Hisazumi et al. (1983) reported the results of focal tumour illumination. Using red light and HpD, they found that tumours greater than 2 cm in diameter were not effectively treated at dosages of 100–250 J/cm^2 and power densities up to 300 mW/cm^2.

Other workers (Benson 1986; Jocham et al. 1986; Shumaker and Hetzel 1987; Williams and Stamp 1988) gave diffuse illuminations using "bulb-tip" optical fibres or intravesical Intralipid. There is no consensus of opinion regarding power density, but a light dose of between 10–70 J/cm^2 produced at least a partial response (reduction of number of tumours by 50%) in up to 83% of patients at 3 months follow-up. Benson (1986) reported that 7 out of 15 patients with pT$_{is}$ had a complete response (eradication of disease and negative cytology) at 6–32 months follow-up; Prout et al. (1987) and Williams and Stamp (1988) also reported promising results in patients with widespread pT$_{is}$.

Side Effects

Skin photosensitisation may be a problem and can last for several weeks. Patients must avoid bright sunlight for several weeks following treatment and take appropriate precautions, including wearing a wide-brimmed hat, gloves and sunglasses when outside.

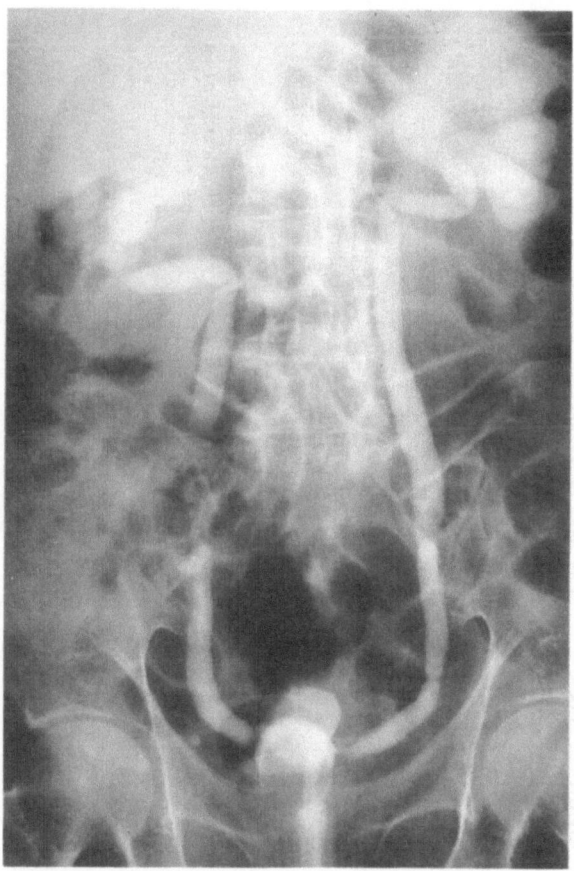

Fig. 6.8. Cystogram of a patient 1 year after PDT. (DHE 2 mg/kg 72 hours before whole bladder illumination at 630 nm. 25 J/cm².)

The commonest reported side effects were dysuria, haematuria, urinary frequency and transient reduction in bladder capacity. In most patients urinary capacity apparently returns to near normal, but a large percentage of the urine volume may reside in dilated refluxing ureters. Three of Harty's 7 patients (Harty et al. 1989) were treated with red light at a dose of 25 J/cm² for "whole bladder" illumination and 100 J/cm² for "focal" treatment, and 1 patient received 25 J/cm² "whole bladder" illumination alone. All these patients developed a severe reduction in bladder capacity, with vesicoureteral reflux and hydronephrosis persistent at 1 year (Figs. 6.8 and 6.9). Cystoscopy showed marked trabeculation of the bladder with fixed dilated ureteric orifices. Bladder biopsies showed severe fibrosis of all layers including muscle (Fig. 6.10). It is not clear whether this is a vascular response to PDT or a direct cytotoxic effect on the smooth muscle cells of the bladder. Nseyo et al. (1987) and Jocham et al. (1986) reported such severe reduction in bladder capacity in some patients that cystectomy was necessary for intractable frequency. Williams has

Table 6.1. Results of PDT in superficial bladder cancer

Author (date)	Patients	Histological stage (UICC 1979)	Sensitisation and dose (mg/kg)	Interval between sensitisation and illumination (h)	Laser and light wavelength (nm)	Type of illumination	Power density (mW/cm²)	Light dose (J/cm²)	Follow-up period (months)	Clinical outcome
Tsuchiya et al. (1983)	8	pT$_a$–pT$_2$	HpD (2.5)	48–72	Arg/dye (635)	Foc	100	120–360	6–18	6 × CR
Hisazumi et al. (1983)	9	pT$_a$–pT$_1$	HpD (2.0–3.2)	48–72	Arg/dye (630)	Foc	150–300	50–300	(3 wks)	Tumours <2 cm diam.: 18 × CR. 6 × PR, 8 × NR. Tumours > 2 cm diam.: 1 × PR. 3 × NR
Hisazumi et al. (1984)	2	pT$_{is}$	HpD (4.0)	48	Arg/dye (630)	WB		10	4	2 × CR
Ohi et al. (1984)	11	pT$_a$–pT$_2$	HpD or Photofrin (2.5)	72	Arg/dye (630)	Foc	100	120	10–22	8 × CR. 3 × NR
Benson (1986)	15 11	pT$_{is}$ (focal)	HpD (2.5–5.0)	3 (+/– repeat at 48 h)	Arg/dye (630)	Foc		150	6–32	7 × CR. 8 × NR
	2 2	pT$_{is}$ (diffuse) pT$_{is}$ + pT$_2$ pT$_{is}$ + pT$_a$	HpD (4.0–5.0)			WB		25–45	3–9	5 × CR. 3 × NR pT$_{is}$ cleared, pT$_a$ + pT$_2$ persisted
Jocham et al. (1986)	5	Superficial + pT$_{is}$	HpD (2.0)			WB		15–70		4 × CR
Shumaker and Hetzel (1987)	15	pT$_a$ + pT$_{is}$	DHE (2.0)	72		WB		25	6–36	11 × CR. 3 × PR. 1 × NR

Table 6.1. (continued)

Author (date)	Patients	Histological stage (UICC 1979)	Sensitisation and dose (mg/kg)	Interval between sensitisation and illumination (h)	Laser and light wavelength (nm)	Type of illumination	Power density (mW/cm²)	Light dose (J/cm²)	Follow-up period (months)	Clinical outcome
Nseyo et al. (1987)	23	pT_a, pT_{is}, pT_1, pT_2, pT_3	DHE (2.0)	72	Arg/dye (630)	WB WB WB + Foc Foc	9–23 10–23 80–400 42–200	10–60 5–60 5–60 WB + 100–200 Foc 50–100	2–12	At 3 mths: 6 × CR, 9 × PR, 6 × NR At 6 mths: 3 × CR
Prout et al. (1987)	19	pT_0, pT_1, pT_{is}	DHE (2.0)	48	Arg/dye (630)	WB + Foc	500–1000	5.5–10 WB + 3 100–200 Foc		9 × CR, 9 × PR, 1 × NR
Harty et al. (1989)	5 2	pT_a, pT_1, pT_{is}	DHE (2.0)	72	Arg/dye (630)	WB + Foc WB		25 WB + 100 Foc 25 WB	12–15	3 × CR, 2 × NR 1 × CR, 1 × NR
Williams and Stamp (1988)	10	pT_a, pT_1 + pT_{is}	DHE (2.0)	72	Au (628) + Cu (514/578)	WB		10–15	3–6	3 × CR, 3 × PR, 3 × NR

Abbreviations: HpD, haematoporphyrin derivative; DHE, dihaematoporphyrin ether (Photofrin II); Arg/dye, argon-ion pumped dye laser; Au, gold vapour laser; Cu, copper vapour laser; Foc, focal illumination of tumour(s); WB, whole bladder illumination; CR, complete response defined as complete eradication of macroscopic + microscopic tumour with negative urine cytology; PR, partial response defined as reduction by > 50% in size or number of tumours without increase in stage or grade; NR, non-response defined as no improvement or worsening of size, numbers, stage or grade of tumours.

found scarred ureteric orifices despite using the less penetrating green light (Williams and Stamp 1988).

Discussion

The treatment parameters in the human studies have been somewhat empirical as there is scant supportive animal data. Nevertheless, despite their small numbers and heterogeneous population, the above reports show that PDT can be successful in treating small superficial tumours and carcinoma in situ. Based on these studies and our experimental work, we suggest that all exophytic tumour should be resected prior to PDT and that invasive tumours should not be treated. We feel that PDT is best suited to treating widespread superficial tumours, carcinoma in situ and areas of "field change" in the urothelium in an attempt to control extensive disease and to destroy microscopic foci rather than focal lesions.

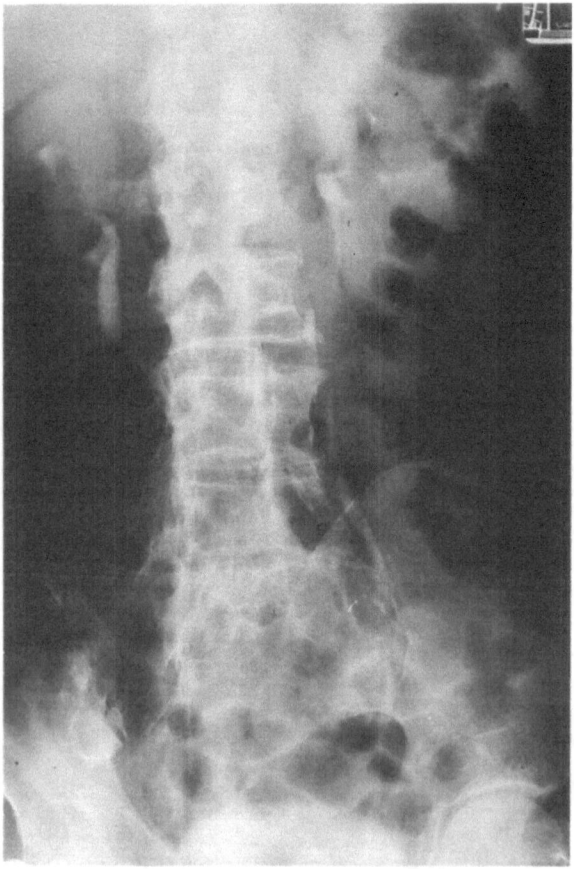

Fig. 6.9. Intravenous urogram of a patient before PDT (a) and 9 months after PDT (b). (DHE 2 mg/kg 72 hours before whole bladder illumination at 630 nm, 25 J/cm².)

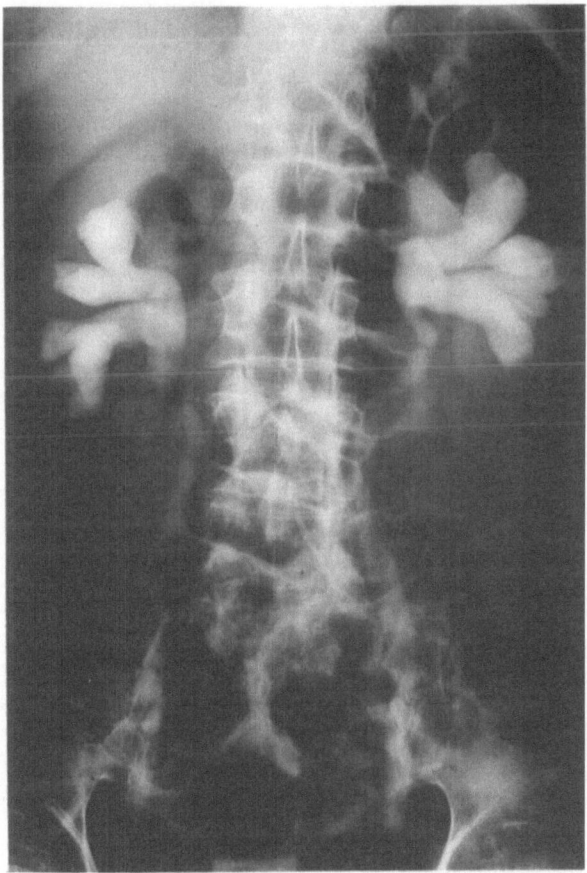

Fig. 6.9b

The severity of the dysuria, frequency and bladder contraction is probably a function of the light dose and wavelength. Red light penetrates tissues more deeply than green light but there are insufficient clinical data at present to compare their relative efficacy and the incidence of side effects.

The St Mary's Hospital PDT Trials

At St. Mary's Hospital in London, we are currently entering patients into phase II clinical trials to determine the efficacy of PDT in patients with pT_a/pT_1 and pT_{is} superficial bladder cancer. These patients will, over a period of at least 1 year, have either failed to maintain a clinical response to conventional therapy or been unable to tolerate the treatment.

The patient undergoes a preliminary cystoscopy and resection of all exophytic tumour; this allows clinical and histological staging of the disease.

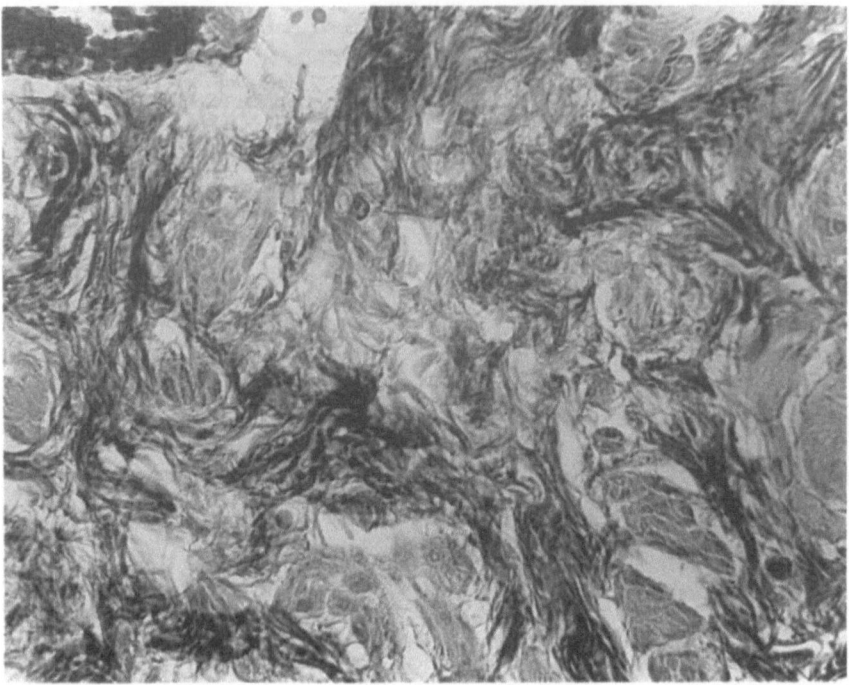

Fig. 6.10. Photomicrograph of biopsy of bladder wall of a patient 1 year after PDT, showing muscle fibrosis. (DHE 2 mg/kg 72 hours before whole bladder illumination at 630 nm, 20 J/cm². Masson trichrome.)

The bladder shape is assessed by per-abdominal ultrasound under deep anaesthesia at maximal distension by 1 m water pressure. The patient is eligible for PDT provided the entry criteria are satisfied, the disease is superficial and the ratio of maximum to minimum internal bladder dimensions is 1.25 : 1.0, i.e. the bladder is virtually spherical.

Informed consent is obtained and the patient given an intravenous injection of HpD (2.5 mg/kg) (Scotia Pharmaceuticals) and nursed in a room with semi-reflective filters on the windows. Twenty-four hours later, with the patient under deep anaesthesia, the bladder is illuminated with green/yellow light from a 25-W copper vapour laser (Oxford Lasers), delivered via a 600-μm optical fibre introduced through a modified cystoscope. The bladder is maximally inflated as above using dilute Intralipid suspension (1 : 500 of 20%). From knowledge of the laser output, the bladder dimensions by ultrasound and the surface area, the whole bladder is treated with 20 J/cm².

Following treatment, the bladder is drained by urethral catheterisation for 24–48 hours. The patient is discharged with a written list of precautions to avoid skin photosensitivity. Repeat cystoscopies are performed at 6 weeks and at regular intervals thereafter, with biopsies of recurrent lesions and four quadrant bladder biopsies. Assessment of treatment is based on clinical and histological changes and on a quality of life questionnaire.

The Future and Conclusions

The search continues for more selective sensitisers (van Lier 1988). These include the meso- and orthoporphyrins (Berenbaum et al. 1986a) and the chlorins (Kessel and Dutton 1984).

The concept of photobleaching may be of relevance (Potter et al. 1987; Mang et al. 1987). This involves sensitising the animal or patient with the lowest concentration of sensitiser that will have a cytotoxic effect. The sensitiser in the normal tissues is rapidly bleached and made inactive by the applied light causing a minimal effect, but where there is sufficient sensitiser (in tumour tissue) the effect is more prolonged resulting in significant damage. Photobleaching has been observed with phthalocyanines (H. Barr and A. McRobert, personal communication).

Control of the light dose within the bladder remains problematic. We are examining new optical fibre tips and exploring methods of moulding them to deliver an isodose to the mucosa of irregular bladders.

In this overview of PDT in superficial bladder cancer we have endeavoured to convey the current concepts of its mechanism, the experimental and clinical data and the areas that warrant further investigation. We believe that PDT can be of value in treating persistent and widespread carcinoma in situ and superficial papillary bladder cancer. However, despite the long history of interest in photosensitisation the development of this therapy is still in its early stages and much remains to be determined.

Acknowledgements. The authors wish to acknowledge the help of Dr. M. C. Berenbaum, Department of Experimental Pathology, St. Mary's Hospital Medical School, London, in the preparation of the manuscript.

References

Auler H, Banzer G (1942) Untersuchungen über die Rolle der Porphyrine bei geschwulstkranken Menschen und Tieren. Z Krebsforsch 53:65–68

Baghdassarian R, Wright MW, Vaughn SA, Berns MW, Martin DG, Wile AG (1985) The use of lipid emulsion as an intravesical medium to disperse light in the potential treatment of bladder tumours. J Urol 133:126–130

Barr H, Tralau CJ, Boulos PB et al. (1987a) The contrasting mechanisms of colonic collagen damage between photodynamic therapy and thermal injury. Photochem Photobiol 46:795–800

Barr H, Tralau CJ, McRobert A et al. (1987b) Photodynamic therapy in the normal rat colon with phthalocyanine sensitisation. Br J Cancer 56:111–118

Bellnier DA, Dougherty TJ (1982) Membrane lysis in Chinese hamster ovary cells with hematoporphyrin derivative plus light. Photochem Photobiol 36:43–47

Ben-Hur E, Rosenthal I (1985) The phthalocyanines: a new class of mammalian cell photosensitizers with a potential for cancer phototherapy. Int J Radiat Biol 47:145–147

Benson RC (1986) Integral photoradiation therapy of multifocal bladder tumors. Eur Urol 12 [Suppl 1]:47–53

Berenbaum MC, Bonnett R, Scourides PA (1982) In vivo activity of the components of haematoporphyrin derivative. Br J Cancer 45:571–581

Berenbaum MC Akande SL, Bonnett R et al. (1986a). Meso-tetra(hydroxyphenyl)porphyrins, a new class of potent tumour photosensitisers with favourable selectivity. Br J Cancer 54:717–725

Berenbaum MC, Hall GW, Hoyes AD (1986b) Cerebral photosensitisation by haematoporphyrin derivative. Evidence for an endothelial site of action. Br J Cancer 53:81–89

Bonnett R, Berenbaum MC (1989) Porphyrins as photosensitising compounds: their chemistry, biology and clinical use. Wiley, Chichester (CIBA Foundation Symposium 146), pp 40–59

Bonnett R, Ridge RJ, Scourides PA, Berenbaum MC (1981) On the nature of haematoporphyrin derivative. J Chem Soc [Perkin 1] 3135–3140

Bown SG, Tralau CJ, Coleridge-Smith PD (1986) Photodynamic therapy with porphyrin and phthalocyanine sensitisation: quantitative studies in normal rat liver. Br J Cancer 5:43–52

Bugelski PJ, Porter CW, Dougherty TJ (1981) Autoradiographic distribution of hematoporphyrin derivative in normal and tumour tissue of the mouse. Cancer Res 41:4606–4612

Diamond I, Granelli SG, McDonagh AF, Neilsen S, Wilson CB, Jaenicke R (1972) Photodynamic therapy of malignant tumours. Lancet ii:1175–1177

Dougherty TJ (1984) Photodynamic therapy (PDT) of malignant tumours. CRC Crit Rev Oncol Hematol 2:83–116

Dougherty TJ (1986) Photosensitization of malignant tumours. Semin Surg Oncol 2:24–37

Dougherty TJ, Grindey GB, Fiel R, Weishaupt KR, Boyle DG (1975) Photoradiation therapy II. Cure of animal tumours with hematoporphyrin and light. J Natl Cancer Inst 55:115–119

Dougherty TJ, Potter WR, Weishaupt R (1984) The structure of the active component of HpD. In: Doiron DR, Gomer CJ (eds) Porphyrin localization and treatment of tumors. Alan R Liss, New York, pp 301–314 (Progress in clinical and biological research vol 170)

Foote CS (1984) Mechanisms of photooxygenation. In: Doiron DR, Gomer CJ (eds) Porphyrin localization and treatment of tumors. Alan R Liss, New York, pp 3–18 (Progress in clinical and biological research vol 170)

Glashan RW (1987) Assessment and treatment of superficial bladder tumours. In: Hendry WF (ed) Recent advances in urology and andrology vol 4. Churchill Livingstone, Edinburgh, pp 187–203

Gomer CJ, Dougherty TJ (1979) Determination of [³H]- and [¹⁴C]-hematoporphyrin derivative distribution in malignant and normal tissue. Cancer Res 39:146–151

Gomer CJ, Razum NJ (1984) Acute skin response in albino mice following porphyrin photosensitisation under oxic and anoxic conditions. Photochem Photobiol 40:435–439

Gomer CJ, Smith DM (1980) Photoinactivation of Chinese hamster cells by haematoporphyrin derivative and red light. Photochem Photobiol 32:341–348

Gregorie HB, Horger EO, Ward JL et al. (1968) Hematoporphyrin derivative fluorescence in malignant neoplasms. Ann Surg 167:820–828

Harty JI, Amin M, Wieman TJ et al. (1989) Complications of whole bladder dihematoporphyrin ether photodynamic therapy. J Urol 141:1341–1346

Henderson BW, Dougherty TJ, Malone PB (1984) Studies of the mechanism of tumour destruction by photoradiation therapy. In: Doiron DR, Gomer CJ (eds) Porphyrin localization and treatment of tumors. Alan R Liss, New York, pp 601–612 (Progress in clinical and biological research vol 170)

Heney NM, Nocks BN, Daly JJ et al. (1982) Ta and T1 bladder carcinoma: location, recurrence and progression. Br J Urol 54:152–157

Hisazumi H, Misaki T, Miyoshi N (1983) Photoradiation therapy of bladder tumours. J Urol 130:685–687

Hisazumi H, Miyoshi N, Naito K et al. (1984) Whole bladder wall photoradiation therapy for carcinoma in situ of the bladder: a preliminary report. J Urol 13:884–887

Jocham D, Staehler G, Chaussy Ch et al. (1984a) Integral dye-laser irradiation of photosensitised bladder tumours with the aid of a light scattering medium. In: Doiron DR, Gomer CJ (eds) Porphyrin localization and treatment of tumors. Alan R Liss, New York, pp 249–256 (Progress in clinical and biological research vol 170)

Jocham D, Staehler G, Unsold E, Chaussy C, Lohrs U (1984b) Dye laser photoradiation therapy of bladder cancer after photosensitization with haematoporphyrin derivative (HpD). Basis for an integral irradiation. In: Andreoni A, Cubeddu R (eds) Porphyrins in tumor phototherapy. Plenum Press, New York, pp 427–438

Jocham D, Schmiedt E, Baumgartner R, Unsold E (1986) Integral laser–photodynamic treatment of multifocal bladder carcinoma photosensitized by hematoporphyrin derivative. Eur Urol 12 [Suppl 1]:43–46

Kelly JF, Snell ME (1976) Hematoporphyrin derivative: a possible aid in the diagnosis and therapy of carcinoma of the bladder. J Urol 115:150–151

Kelly JF, Snell ME, Berenbaum MC (1975) Photodynamic destruction of human bladder carcinoma. Br J Cancer 31:237-245

Kessel D (1986) Proposed structure of the tumour-localizing fraction of HpD (hematoporphyrin derivative). Photochem Photobiol 44:193-196

Kessel D, Dutton CJ (1984) Photodynamic effects: porphyrin vs. chlorin. Photochem Photobiol 40:403-405

Lin C, Bellnier DA, Fujime M, Prout GR (1984) HpD photodetection of bladder carcinoma. In: Doiron DR, Gomer CJ (eds) Porphyrin localization and treatment of tumors. Alan R Liss, New York, pp 187-199 (Progress in clinical and biological research vol 170)

Lipson RL, Baldes EJ, Olsen AM (1961) The use of a derivative of hematoporphyrin in tumour detection. J Natl Cancer Inst 26:1-11

Lipson RL, Gray MJ, Baldes EJ (1967) Hematoporphyrin derivative for detection and management of cancer. In: Harris RCJ (ed) Proceedings of the ninth international cancer congress. Springer, Berlin Heidelberg New York

Lottmann H (1987) Thèse Médecin, Paris

Lottmann H, Harty JI, Tralau CJ, Bown SG (1988) The effect of photodynamic therapy with phthalocyanine sensitization on the strength and compliance of the normal rat bladder. Paper presented at the sixth annual meeting of the British Medical Laser Association, London

Malik Z, Djaldetti M (1980) Destruction of erythroleukaemia, myelocytic leukaemia and Burkitt lymphoma cells by photoactivated protoporphyrin. Int J Cancer 26:495-500

Mang TS, Dougherty TJ, Potter WR, Boyle DG, Somer S, Moan J (1987) Photobleaching of porphyrin used in photodynamic therapy and implications for therapy. Photochem Photobiol 45:501-506

Moan J (1986) Porphyrin-sensitized photodynamic inactivation of cells: a review. Lasers Med Sci 1:5-12

Nseyo UO, Dougherty TJ, Boyle DG et al. (1985) Experimental photodynamic treatment of canine bladder. J Urol 133:311-315

Nseyo UO, Dougherty TJ, Sullivan L (1987) Experimental photodynamic treatment of resistant lower urinary tract carcinoma. Cancer 60:3113-3119

Ohi T, Kato H, Tsuchiya A (1984) Photoradiation therapy with hematoporphyrin derivative and an argon dye laser of bladder carcinoma. In: Adreoni A, Cubeddu R (eds) Porphyrins in tumor phototherapy. Plenum Press, New York, pp 439-446

OPCS (1988) Cancer statistics registrations. Cases of diagnosed cancer registered in England and Wales 1984. HMSO, London (Office of Population Censuses and Surveys series MB1, no 16)

Plail RO, Berenbaum MC, Snell MS (1988) Histological effects of photodynamic therapy on normal and neoplastic rat bladder sensitized with haematoporphyrin derivative and treated with light at 511 and 578 nm. Paper presented at the British Association of Urological Surgeons annual meeting, Buxton, June 1988

Policard A (1924) Etude sur les aspects offerts par des tumeurs éxperimentales examinées à la luminere de Wood. C R Soc Biol (Paris) 91:1423-1424

Potter WR, Mang TS, Dougherty TJ (1987) The theory of photodynamic dosimetry: consequences of photodestruction of the sensitizer. Photochem Photobiol 46:97-101

Prout GJ Jr, Lin C, Benson RC Jr et al. (1987) Photodynamic therapy with hematoporphyrin derivative in the treatment of superficial transitional cell carcinoma of the bladder. N Engl J Med 317:1251-1255

Raab O (1900) Ueber die Wirkung fluoreszierender Stoffe auf Influsorien. Z Biol 39:524-546

Selman SH, Kreimer-Birnbaum M, Klaunig JE, Goldblatt PJ, Keck RW, Britton SL (1984) Blood flow in transplantable bladder tumours treated with hematoporphyrin derivative and light. Cancer Res 44:1924-1927

Selman SH, Goldblatt PJ, Klaunig JE, Keck RW, Kreimer-Birnbaum M (1985) Localisation of hematoporphyrin derivative in injured bladder mucosa. An experimental study. J Urol 133:1104-1107

Severs NJ, Barnes SH, Wright R, Hicks RM (1982) Induction of bladder cancer in rats by fractionated intravesicular doses of N-methyl-N-nitrosurea. B J Cancer 45:337-351

Shumaker PB, Hetzel FW (1987) Clinical laser photodynamic therapy in the treatment of bladder carcinoma. Photochem Photobiol 46:899-909

Spikes JD (1984) Photobiology of porphyrins. In: Doiron DR, Gomer CJ (eds) Porphyrin localization and treatment of tumours. Alan R Liss, New York, pp 19-39 (Progress in clinical and biological research vol 170)

Star WM, Marijnissen JPA, van den Berg-Blok AE, Reinhold HS (1984) Destructive effect of photoradiation on the microcirculation of a rat mammary tumour growing in "sandwich" observation chambers. In: Doiron DR. Gomer CJ (eds) Porphyrin localization and treatment of tumors. Alan R Liss. pp 637–645 (Progress in clinical and biological research vol 170)

Star WM. Marijnissen HPA. Jansen H. Keijzer M. van Gemert MJC (1987) Light dosimetry for photodynamic therapy by whole bladder wall irradiation. Photochem. Photobiol 46:619–624

Svaasand L (1985) Photodynamic and photohyperthermic response of malignant tumours. Med Phys 12:455–461

Tappeiner H. Jesionek A (1903) Therapeutische Versuche mit fluoreszierenden Stoffen. MWWR 2:2040–2044

Tsuchiya A. Obara N. Miwa M. Ohi T. Kato H. Hayata Y (1983) Hematoporphyrin derivative and laser photoradiation in the diagnosis and treatment of bladder cancer. J Urol 130:79–82

van Gemert JC. Berenbaum MC. Gijsbers GHM (1985) Wavelength and light-dose dependence in tumour phototherapy with hematoporphyrin derivative. Br J Cancer 52:43–49

van Lier JE (1988) New sensitizers for photodynamic therapy of cancer. Light in Biology and Medicine 1:133–141

Weishaupt KR. Gomer CL. Dougherty TJ (1976) Identification of singlet oxygen as the cytotoxic agent in photoinactivation of a murine tumour. Cancer Res 36:2326–2329

Williams JL. Stamp J (1988) Photodynamic therapy in the treatment of multiple superficial tumours of the bladder. Presentation at the British Association of Urological Surgeons annual meeting. Buxton. June 1988

Chapter 7

Interstitial Hyperthermia of the Prostate

A. C. Steger and T. A. McNicholas

Historical Background

Hyperthermia involves the use of heat to treat malignancy. There are references to the therapeutic use of heat in ancient Egypt (Edwin Smith surgical papyrus, *c.* 1700 BC) and Hippocrates stated that "diseases not cured by drugs are cured by surgery, conditions not cured by surgery are cured by cauterisation and conditions not cured by cauterisation should be considered incurable". It was not, however, until the end of the nineteenth century that the scientific study of the effect of heat on malignancies was begun. The first observations were in Germany in the 1860s, but Coley (Coley 1894) in America treated patients with sarcomas by injecting a mixture of bacterial toxins and raising the body temperature to 41–42 °C for 4–6 hours. The results of this work were a demonstrable response in over half of those treated and an increase in expected survival in 20%. After this, interest in hyperthermia fell with the introduction and use of radiotherapy for treating cancers. Since the 1950s there has been an increased interest in the possible use of hyperthermia to treat cancer, and a vast amount of experimental work to investigate the mechanisms by which heat has its effect and the outcome of clinical applications (Hahn 1982).

In the temperature range 41–45 °C there is some degree of selectivity in the effect of heat on normal and malignant tissues, with the latter being somewhat more sensitive. Above 50 °C (and probably above 45 °C) this selectivity is lost, and there is an equal thermal effect on normal and malignant tissue. For these reasons research on hyperthermia and its clinical application has focused on the temperature range 41–45 °C.

There is some evidence to suggest that there is a difference in the cellular response of a normal and a malignant cell to thermal energy. The relationship between temperature and the time for which the tissue is exposed to the heat is crucial. The Arrhenius relationship says that for each degree (Celsius) of temperature rise there is a halving of the time required to achieve cell death (Overgaard and Suit 1979); this relationship broadly applies to all tissues and methods of heat delivery.

There are two types of mechanism by which thermal energy has an effect on a tumour: the specifically cellular and those affecting the tumour as a whole. The effect on the cell is probably by damage to intracellular proteins and lipoprotein structures. The activation energy required to cause hyperthermic cell damage is very similar to that required for protein damage, being 150 kcal/mol (Henriques 1947). The effect of heat on tumour is due to a number of factors including vascular shut-down in tumour circulation, the opening up of vessels in normal tissue around the tumour with a vascular "steal" effect, acidosis and an increase in interstitial fluid. These all result in reduced blood flow and low tumour pH and glucose level, with subsequent cell death within the tumour.

A large number of mechanisms for delivering heat to tumours have been tried, from steam baths and hot air convectors in the 1930s and 1940s to the current preference for microwave and radiofrequency wavelengths. Other methods include the isolated heating of an organ or limb, and whole-body hyperthermia. Whilst probably few patients have been cured of a malignancy with hyperthermic treatment there is good evidence that reduction in tumour growth rate and size and an increase in survival can be achieved when hyperthermia is used in conjunction with radiotherapy and chemotherapy (Falk et al. 1986).

The disadvantage of all the current methods of delivering thermal energy is that it is difficult to maintain the required temperature for an adequate time to the whole of the relevant tissue volume, so as to ensure complete thermal damage of the target, while at the same time avoiding excessive damage to surrounding normal tissues. This is why most clinical work has dealt with skin tumours, which are readily accessible, and also why hyperthermic treatment requires a number of repeat sessions to try to achieve adequate thermal damage of the target tumour.

Interstitial therapy, that is the insertion of the chosen energy delivery source into the tissue to be treated, offers the possibility of more controlled tumour heating. The problems of the application of existing hyperthermic methods still remain. For these reasons the use of interstitial laser energy delivered by a small-calibre fibre placed into tumour tissue is most attractive.

Early Studies on Interstitial Therapy

Urological interest has concentrated on the bladder and particularly the prostate, and there has been a renewed burst of activity on the microwave front recently. Yerushalmi (1988) described a 2.45-GHz microwave system for treating prostate cancer that uses a transrectal applicator with a cooling system to avoid thermal damage to the rectal wall. A system of temperature measurement from within the prostatic urethra and a computerised sensing system with a feedback loop is designed to prevent excessive heating that would damage the rectum and distal sphincter mechanism. This method is intended to achieve the traditional hyperthermic temperature range of 43–44°C and therefore to utilise any increased sensitivity of malignant tissue to raised temperatures.

A number of patients were treated by this system but also received radio-therapy. Some patients survived for 20–40 months, but there was no correlation between local recurrence and initial or complete or partial response and metastatic spread. It is therefore difficult to be certain of the effect of the hyperthermic treatment on the disease reported here. Patients did not have any side effects that could be attributed to the hyperthermia itself. However, in an experimental study on the rabbit prostate by the same group, the same micro-wave system and similar temperatures produced no histological evidence of hyperthermic damage at all (Yerushalmi et al. 1983).

One major problem with microwave techniques such as this would appear to be that the heat deposition is not well controlled or well localised to the most abnormal areas. There has been little work on ultrasound or radiofrequency hyperthermia in the urological environment, though the relatively simpler con-cept of raising bladder wall temperature by irrigation with warm solutions has been explored by several groups (Hall et al. 1974; Jacob et al. 1982).

Obviously a laser could be used as the energy source, the light being con-ducted through a flexible fibre which could pass through a fine needle into the area of abnormal tissue. The exact positioning of the needle can be relatively easily achieved using ultrasound techniques. The use of the YAG laser and a fibre-optic transmission system for this purpose was suggested by Bown in 1983. Since that time Bown and co-workers have explored this possibility and interest has spread widely. Hashimoto et al. (1985) described what appears to be the first clinical application of Bown's suggested technique. Under ultra-sonic imaging a tumour of the liver was identified, its volume calculated and a quartz glass fibre inserted into its centre. Using a continuous wave YAG laser at a power of 15 W, energy was then administered according to a protocol of 100 J/cm^3 of tumour.

Matthewson et al. (1987) placed single fibres in rat liver and described areas of coagulation of approximately 15 mm diameter surrounding the YAG laser fibre. Subsequent studies in larger animals, particularly the dog, have con-firmed that single fibres can cause homogeneous areas of necrosis in the canine pancreas and liver varying from 12 to 15 mm in maximum diameter (Steger et al. 1988). Rather larger lesions could be created using multiple fibres (Steger et al. 1988). Workers from the same unit (Matthewson et al. 1989) have implanted fibres in rats bearing a transplantable fibrosarcoma and have treated cohorts of rats with varying combinations of power and exposure times; there have been a range of effects on the target tumours. Most recently early clinical experience has been reported (Steger et al. 1989).

The lesions described above were produced using "energy doses" of between 675 and 1000 J. This suggests there is a threshold "dose" of laser energy which can cause a fairly predictable amount of thermal necrosis in a variety of organs. It is not entirely clear why such relatively homogeneous results should be found in such different organs and indeed in different animals. The pros-tate, pancreas and liver differ with regard to optical density (colour) and there-fore light penetration. They also have different thermal diffusion and blood flow characteristics, all of which should cause an alteration of the energy absorbed per unit volume of tissue.

Godlewski et al. (1988) described a YAG laser interstitial method using a 5-

mm diameter probe to carry a fibre to the target tissue but employing a much higher power (80 W) for a shorter period (10 seconds) – similar parameters to those used in traditional endoscopic practice. They produced 12–18-mm diameter lesions in pig liver with marked central cavitation and charring. Despite the much higher powers used the temperatures measured at 1 cm from laser source were very similar to those found in the low-power studies of Bown's groups.

Experimental Studies in Prostatic Interstitial Hyperthermia

As discussed in Chapter 4, prostate cancer remains a challenge to the urologist. The increasingly sophisticated imaging methods available, particularly ultrasound, allow the detection of suspicious areas which can then be biopsied much more precisely than hitherto (Fig. 7.1). And it is this very success of ultrasound imaging and ultrasound-guided biopsy techniques for the small prostatic tumours that has served to reawaken interest in their surgical treatment. McNeal et al. (1986) have, by virtue of precise pathological studies of large numbers of males, elegantly described the relationship between tumour volume and progression of disease and metastasis. Their studies suggest that lesions of small volume (below 1 ml) correlate with a very low risk of extraprostatic spread. It is of interest that the same characteristics are also being found for breast cancer (Forrest 1989).

Bearing in mind the ability to image and place a biopsy needle within such lesions, the exciting possibility therefore arises of using these relatively common-place needling techniques to place an energy source within the abnormal area

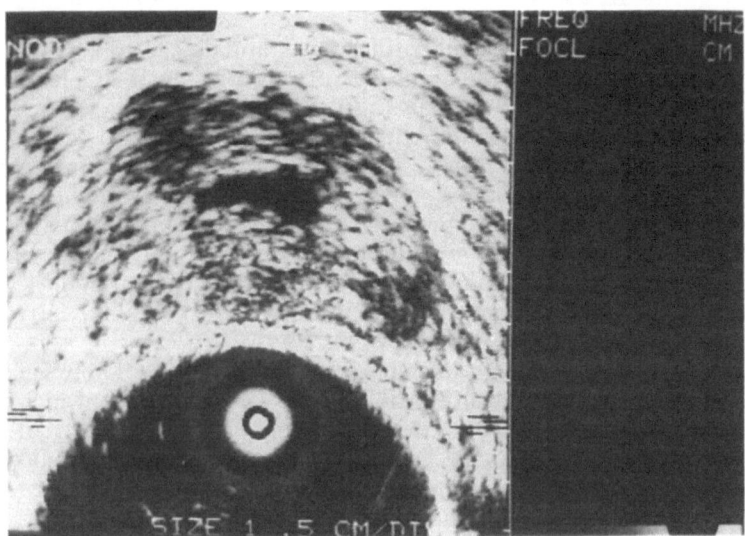

Fig. 7.1. Axial transrectal ultrasound (TRUS) of prostate showing small echopenic area at left base of prostate characteristic of adenocarcinoma and subsequently biopsy proven on TRUS-guided biopsy. (Courtesy of S. St.C. Carter and C. Charig. Institute of Urology.)

so as to cause local tissue destruction. However, any such effect would have to be applied within carefully controlled and, ideally, reasonably predictable limits.

We have been assessing the practicalities of applying the low-power YAG laser interstitial technique to the prostate since 1986 (McNicholas et al. 1988). The beagle prostate is an available model for testing whether these fibres can be implanted within the prostate and for determining the response of the gland to energy deposition. The gland was exposed through a suprapubic midline incision and mobilised. Either single (400 μm) or multiple (100 μm) fibres were implanted through the anterolateral surface of the gland on each side. Low-power laser energy at 1 or 1.5 W was applied over a time period to supply a range of energy doses from 500 J to 1500 J to a series of prostates and the results assessed between 1 and 120 days later.

For this method to be successful it is necessary to have a laser capable of reliably producing such low powers in a stable manner. New clinical models may be able to provide these low powers, but the output range of a laser should be checked before purchase.

Thermocouple measurements made from points adjacent to the fibre tip recorded temperatures approaching 90°C. A distinct temperature gradient was measured by successively more peripherally placed thermocouples until at a point approximately 10 mm from the fibre tip the temperature was between 36°C and 38°C. This correlated with the margins of the necrotic area seen at post-mortem. These temperatures near the fibre tip are obviously higher than those encountered in traditional hyperthermia. We accept that the method does not seek to benefit to any great degree from the relative heat sensitivity of tumour tissue. Rather it exerts an effect by precisely but gradually supplying a large volume of energy as heat, causing the tissue temperature to rise well above hyperthermic levels and into the range where there is no doubt that cell death will occur, whether those cells be normal or malignant.

A problem encountered in most other hyperthermic methods is that of ensuring the accurate delivery of adequate amounts of energy without damaging adjacent tissue through which either the energy itself or the energy delivery mechanism has to pass. This experimental technique allows the use of extremely fine fibres which will pass easily through the calibre of needles routinely used for biopsy or, indeed, through smaller-bore needles if necessary (i.e. if it were necessary to use multiple fibres to treat a larger area or to allow a particular lesion to be "surrounded").

Though high, the temperatures generated are very localised. If the operator can see (ultrasonically) the end of the fibre he can assess where the region of high temperature will be. Experimental and clinical work in other organs suggests that the actual heating process can be observed ultrasonically, an area of mixed hyperechoic signal being seen (Steger et al. 1989). This does not detract from the need to develop sensitive thermometry methods to accompany the safe use of interstitial laser hyperthermia. Clinical trial of interstitial laser hyperthermia for superficial (breast tumour secondaries) and deeply situated targets (pancreatic and hepatic tumours) (Steger et al. 1989) has not revealed discomfort when these temperatures have been achieved.

Our results showed that lesions could reliably be produced and their size varied according to the total energy dose. There appeared to be a threshold of approximately 650–700 J below which tissue necrosis was negligible. Above that threshold and up to 1500 J a lesion of approximately 15 mm maximum

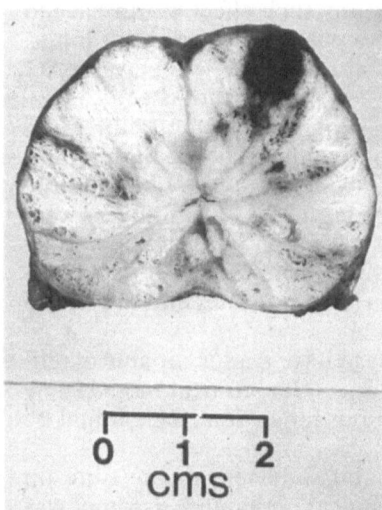

Fig. 7.2. Specimen 2 weeks after interstitial YAG laser coagulation showing well-defined necrotic area.

diameter resulted. This was characteristically well-demarcated (Fig. 7.2) with an abrupt change from abnormal to normal tissue on histological examination as shown on Fig. 7.3. At 2 months after treatment healing was by fibrosis and cystic degeneration.

The animals suffered no ill effects from the implantation with the exception of one, in which the fibres were placed inadvertently close to the urethra. This caused a urinary fistula between the needle track, the cavity where the maximal thermal injury had resulted in a large area of necrosis and the perforated urethra.

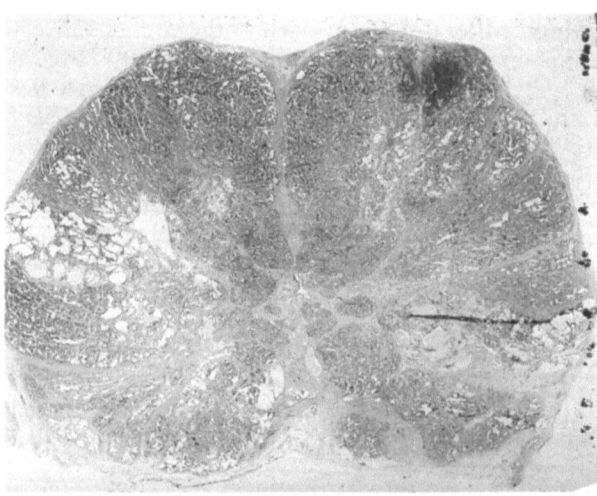

Fig. 7.3. Same specimen 2 weeks after interstitial YAG coagulation showing well-defined area of coagulative necrosis on pathological whole mount. (Courtesy of Mr. D. Butcher and Dr. M. C. Parkinson. Institute of Urology.)

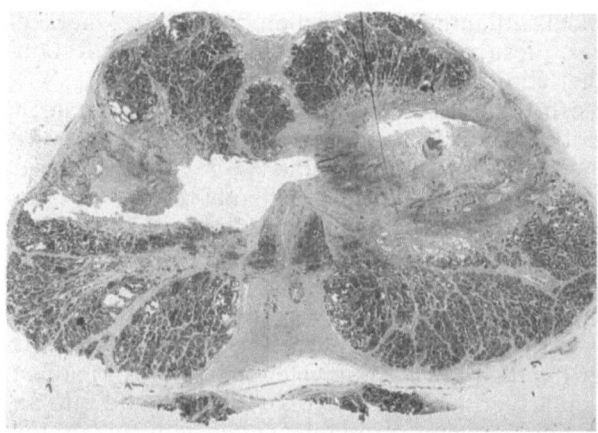

Fig. 7.4. Canine prostate with larger volume lesion shown on ultrasound.

Ultrasound in our hands was not particularly successful in guiding the fibres into the prostate when we attempted a percutaneous perineal approach, but did show clearly echopenic areas corresponding to the cystic lesions found when the prostates were scanned in vitro post-mortem at six weeks. Other ultrasonically detectable changes corresponded to the area of necrosis seen on specimens when sectioned (Figs. 7.4, 7.5) at earlier stages.

Overall these experimental studies suggested that lesions of approximately the size of small localised early prostatic cancers found in clinical practice could be destroyed *in situ* by an interstitial implantation technique.

Similar animal experiments using multiple fibres showed that larger volume areas could be destroyed in the same manner. Larger lesions were created but with an increased risk of the margin of necrosis transgressing the urethra. This

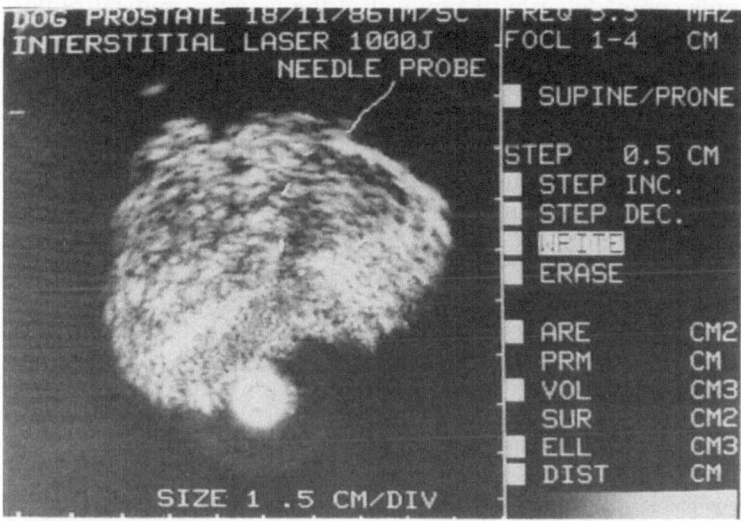

Fig. 7.5. Same canine prostate with large volume lesion (at 2 weeks after treatment).

led to a much more marked inflammatory reaction and more marked cavitation of the necrotic area, presumably related to superimposed infection from the urinary tract. Further clinical studies are under way.

Littrup et al. (1988) have recently described the ablation of canine prostate in a similar manner to that described above, but using powers between 15 and 60 W for 5 seconds, giving total energy doses between 75 and 300 J. They compared the effects of percutaneous injection of absolute ethanol or YAG laser hyperthermia, both via a fibre inserted under transrectal ultrasound guidance. Their results are very similar to ours, the tissue effects being much better controlled when produced by the laser than with ethanol.

Whilst Littrup et al.'s 5-second treatment times seem at first sight attractive compared with the 600–1500-second exposures of our lower-power method, it is our impression that a slower treatment will give greater opportunity to adjust the fibre(s) position(s), particularly if the laser effect is seen to extend into an undesirable area. Multiple fibre systems available either now or in the foreseeable future cannot cope with the high powers used by Littrup et al. and, indeed, YAG lasers are not available that will produce enough laser power to give 60 W down each of four fibres as we use experimentally.

Conclusion

The real significance of laser interstitial hyperthermia cannot be assessed yet, but it does provide the possibility of treating the lesions that can already be seen and accurately biopsied in clinical practice. The exciting possibility arises of using these same methods with the addition of the coagulating thermal effect of the YAG laser to create localised necrosis in those abnormal areas.

The technique may prove an alternative treatment for small focal prostatic cancers that avoids complete surgical removal of the gland or radical radiotherapy. It may have the advantage of being repeatable, and this may be particularly important where the extent of the tumour has been underestimated or if tumours recur subsequently. Either of these possibilities may become apparent, particularly with increased sensitivity of future ultrasound scanning techniques. Finally, the destruction of focal tumour mass may render low volume, diffuse disease elsewhere within the gland treatable by radiotherapy or by the application of PDT techniques using the same interstitial (multiple) fibre technique after the administration of a photosensitiser.

References

Bown SG (1983) Phototherapy of tumours. World J Surg 7:700–709
Coley WB (1894) Treatment of inoperable malignant tumours with the toxins of erysipelas and the *Bacillus prodigus*. Am J Med Sci 108(1):50–66

Falk RE, Newhook L, Moffat FL et al. (1986) Thermochemotherapy for unresectable hepatic metastases. In: Herfarth C, Schlag P, Hohenberger P (eds) Therapeutic strategies in primary and metastatic liver cancer. Springer, Berlin Heidelberg New York, pp 315-20 (Recent results in cancer research vol 100)

Forrest APM (1989) Tamoxifen comes of age. Br J Surg 76:325-326

Godlewski G, Sambuc P, Eledjam JJ, Rouy S, Pignodel C, Ould-Said A, Bourgeois JM (1988) A new device for inducing deep localised vaporisation in liver with the Nd-YAG laser. Lasers Med Sci 3:111-117

Hahn GM (1982) Hyperthermia and cancer. Plenum Press, New York

Hall RR, Schade ROK, Swinney J (1974) Effects of hyperthermia on bladder cancer. Br Med J ii:593-4

Hashimoto D, Takami M, Idezuki Y (1985) In depth radiation therapy by YAG laser for malignant tumours in the liver under ultrasonic imaging. Gastroenterology 88:1663

Henriques FC (1947) Studies of thermal injury. V. The predictability and the significance of thermally induced rate processes leading to irreversible epidermal injury. Arch Pathol 43:489-502

Jacob J, Hindmarsh JR, Ludgate CM, Chisholm GD (1982) Observations on the ultrastructure of human urothelium: the response of normal bladders of elderly subjects to hyperthermia. Urol Res 10:227-237

Littrup PJ, Lee F, Borlaza GS, Sacknoff EJ (1988) Percutaneous ablation of canine prostate using transrectal ultrasound guidance, absolute ethanol and Nd:YAG laser. Invest Radiol 23:734-739

Matthewson K, Coleridge-Smith P, O'Sullivan JP, Northfield TC, Bown SG (1987) Biological effects of intrahepatic Nd-YAG laser photocoagulation in the rat. Gastroenterology 93:550-557

Matthewson K, Barr H, Tralau C, Bown SG (1989) Low power interstitial Nd-YAG laser photocoagulation: studies in a transplantable fibrosarcoma. Br J Surg 76:378-381

McNeal JE, Kindrachuk RA, Freiha FS, Bostwick DG, Redwine EA, Stamey TA (1986) Patterns of progression in prostate cancer. Lancet i:60-63

McNicholas TA, Steger AC, Charig C, Bown SG (1988) Interstitial YAG laser coagulation of the prostate. Lasers Med Sci 3 [abstracts issue] abstr 446

Overgaard J, Suit HD (1979) Time-temperature relationships in hyperthermic treatment of malignant and normal tissue in vivo. Cancer Res 39:3248-3253

Steger AC, Barr H, Bown SG, Clark CG (1987) Experimental studies on low power laser interstitial hyperthermia for pancreatic carcinoma. Gut 28:A1382

Steger AC, Bown SG, Clarke CG (1988) Interstitial laser hyperthermia: studies in the normal liver. Br J Surg 75:598

Steger AC, Lees WR, Walmsley K, Bown SG (1989) Interstitial laser hyperthermia: a new approach to local destruction of tumours. Br Med J 299:362-365

Yerushalmi A (1988) Localised non-invasive deep microwave hyperthermia for the treatment of prostatic tumours: the first 5 years. In: Issels RD, Wilmanns W (eds) Application of hyperthermia in the treatment of cancer. Springer, Berlin Heidelberg New York, pp 141-146 (Recent results in cancer research vol 107)

Yerushalmi A, Shepirer Z, Hod I, Gottefeld F, Bass DD (1983) Normal tissue response to localised deep microwave hyperthermia in the rabbit's prostate: a preclinical study. Int J Radiat Oncol Biol Phys 9:77-82

Chapter 8

Laser Lithotripsy

G. M. Watson

The pulsed dye laser was the first laser to be used for stone fragmentation in clinical practice, and to date it has been employed in the treatment of over 2000 patients world-wide. Other laser systems have also been developed, using Q-switched neodymium yttrium aluminium garnet (YAG) technology. In this chapter the development of the pulsed dye laser for stone fragmentation is described and compared with YAG technology. The techniques of laser stone fragmentation are then explained and compared with methods of electro-hydraulic and ultrasonic stone fragmentation.

Historical Background

In 1968 Mulvaney and Beck used a ruby laser in an attempt to fragment calculi. The ruby laser was the first to become available and interestingly was closer to the optimum than any other system to be tried until 1984. It delivers light at 690 nm and at pulse durations ranging from 10 microseconds at low energy to 800 microseconds at maximum energy output. Mulvaney and Beck used this laser through solid glass rods. Smaller-calibre fibres would have been much more effective, but as it was they were able to fragment certain calculi by using very high energies. Subsequently the conventional medical lasers were assessed. Tanahashi et al. (1981) and Pensel et al. (1981) described using the continuous wave CO_2 and YAG lasers on calculi. Continuous wave lasers have a thermal action alone on calculi. The CO_2 laser is not as yet suitable for urological endoscopic applications for reasons discussed in Chap. 5. The continuous wave YAG laser merely heats up calculi and should never be used clinically for stone fragmentation.

Fair, in 1978, described how it was possible to confine a very thin layer of metal which under the action of the Q-switched pulsed laser generated a shockwave. He constructed a capsule in which he placed this confined metallic layer and the stone. When he delivered a laser pulse to a window in the capsule he was able to fragment the enclosed stone. This was an important experiment because it showed that pulsed lasers could be used to generate shockwaves sufficient to fragment calculi. However, his indirect method of generating a shockwave using a thin layer of confined metal could never be evolved into a system for clinical use.

Pensel et al. (1981) tried using single giant Q-switched lasers directly on calculi without any intervening fibre and were able to fragment certain fragile stones. Watson et al. (1983) showed that trains of smaller-energy Q-switched pulses slowly eroded the surface of the stone even when there was no apparent effect with the single giant Q-switched pulse. Watson then went on to evaluate the 100-microsecond pulsed YAG laser delivered through a fibre. This system could fragment certain dark and fragile calculi when the fibre was placed against the stone surface under water. Although the parameters used were far from ideal, this was the first successful attempt using a laser system which could be tested endoscopically. Watson did not consider it satisfactory, however, because there was a distinct risk of tissue injury due to the high energies produced. Interestingly, though, the fibre withstood prolonged contact with the stone – in contrast to the continuous wave YAG laser, where the tip of the fibre rapidly became overheated and ceased to transmit the laser energy.

Spectroscopy

The basic principle of laser action is that it only has an effect where it is absorbed (although thermal diffusion from absorbing areas can cause secondary effects). In the case of pulsed lasers at very short pulse durations the power density is so great that there can be ionisation of the medium, the free electrons which are liberated in the presence of this high power density of photons causing the release of further electrons. This electron avalanche, or "plasma", absorbs any further laser energy very intensely. Q-switched laser pulses with pulse durations in the region of 10 nanoseconds can form these ionisation plasmas with absent or minimal absorption. Longer pulse durations, including microsecond pulses, require much more absorption for plasma formation.

Spectroscopy on discs of stones was performed using a Beckman spectrophotometer and integrating sphere to correct for the intense scattering. A schematic representation for a typical calculus is shown in Fig. 8.1, where the percentage absorption is plotted against wavelength from 250 to 2500 nm. It can be seen that absorption is extremely dependent on the wavelength of the laser. Therefore, the action of any laser with a pulse duration of 1 microsecond or longer will be governed by this absorption curve. The action of these lasers on tissue will also be governed by these same principles. In Fig. 8.1. the absorption characteristics for normal ureter and for hyperaemic ureter are also shown.

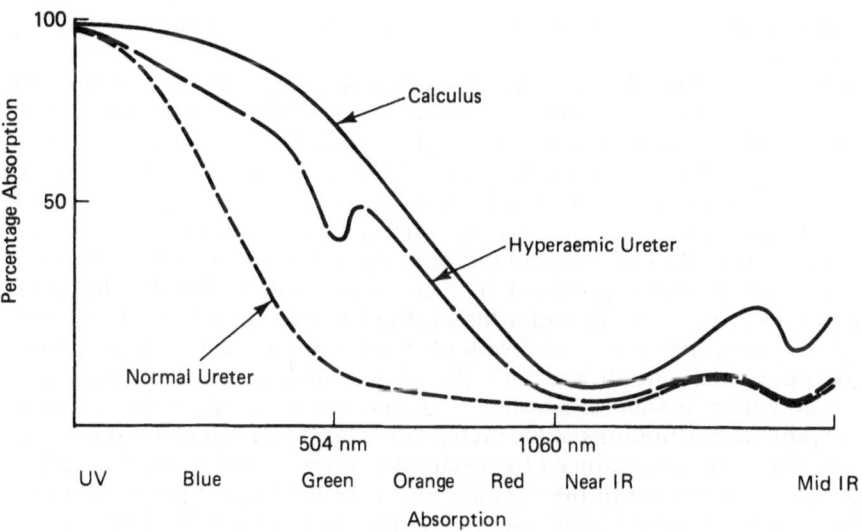

Fig. 8.1. Absorption of laser energy by calculus and water across the range of wavelengths 250–2500 nm. (By courtesy of the Institute of Urology.)

Laser Systems for Stone Fragmentation

Pulsed Dye Lasers

Pulsed dye lasers were tested at the Wellman Laboratories of the Massachusetts General Hospital (Watson et al. 1987a) It was possible to vary the wavelength of the lasers from 450 to 590 nm and the pulse duration from 1 to 360 microseconds. The output from the pulsed dye lasers could be transmitted through fibres varying from 200 μm to 1 mm in diameter. It was therefore possible to perform a full parametric study during which two parameters were kept constant and the remaining parameter varied in order to study its influence.

The energy threshold for fragmentation was found to vary with different laser wavelengths, the threshold being lowest at 540 nm, intermediate at 504 nm and highest at 577 nm. The threshold therefore became higher as absorption dropped off. The threshold also became higher with increasing pulse duration. When fibre diameter was varied there was a very dramatic reduction in the threshold as the diameter was reduced. When the threshold was plotted against the surface area of the fibre, the relationship was approximately linear. Thus with pulsed lasers where the pulse duration was a microsecond or longer, fragmentation was seen to be dependent on absorption and the power density of the laser irradiation at the stone surface.

Although the most efficient parameters for stone fragmentation were found to be a wavelength of 450 nm or less, a pulse duration of 1 microsecond or shorter and a fibre diameter of 200 μm or less, various compromises have been made in order to achieve the most clinically useful system. For example, it can be seen from Fig. 8.1. that the wavelength at which there is the maximum differential absorption of laser energy is 504 nm both for the normal ureter and the hyperaemic ureter.

The prototype clinical pulsed dye laser was therefore set at the following parameters: a wavelength of 504 nm, a pulse duration of 1 microsecond, a fibre diameter of 200 μm and a repetition rate of up to 20 Hz. The laser energy was initially set at 30 mJ and a repetition rate of 10 Hz. If the stone was resistant, then the laser energy was increased in 10-mJ increments up to a maximum of 60 mJ. When the fibre was touching the surface of a typical ureteric calculus under water, then the calculus would break up in a very controlled manner. The surrounding ureter, provided it is not hyperaemic, absorbs the laser irradiation extremely poorly and a burst of pulses can be delivered with the laser fibre against the ureteric wall with no effect whatsoever. Eventually, however, purpura would result and then the effect would be as for hyperaemic ureter, where there is some absorption and therefore some effect. It is possible to cause pinhole perforations of the ureter with a laser – in complete contrast to the large fenestrations produced by discharges of an electro-hydraulic probe.

A good demonstration of the selective effects of the laser is provided when the laser is used on an egg shell. The crystalline shell absorbs the laser energy and there is a characteristic noise and shockwave production. The thin protein membrane underneath the shell, however, does not absorb the laser energy and there is no noise and no shockwave when the laser energy is delivered to this surface. The laser therefore removes the shell leaving the thin protein layer underneath intact, giving a very convincing demonstration of selective photofragmentation.

The pulsed dye laser system lends itself extremely well to ureteroscopic stone fragmentation. The laser is simply placed on the stone surface and the stone can be fragmented with minimal effect to the surrounding ureter. The majority of stones are fragmented extremely efficiently and any relatively large particles can be broken down to fine grit because of the precise application of the laser energy. Calcium oxalate dihydrate, struvite and urate stones are broken down particularly well. Calcium oxalate monohydrate and brushite calculi, however, are very much harder to break down (as they are for any fragmentation mechanism) and the laser merely cleaves them into larger particles which may require basket removal.

The mechanism by which the laser fragments calculi has been shown very elegantly by Teng et al. (1987) to be due to plasma formation at the stone surface. In order for the plasma to effect fragmentation, it requires confinement by all the surrounding fluid. In contrast to the plasma production by a Q-switched pulsed YAG laser, plasma is only produced by pulsed dye lasers with microsecond pulse durations when there is sufficient absorption to initiate it. It is thought to be a thermionic plasma, initiated by very intense heating of a tiny

Table 8.1. The peak power density of the pulsed dye laser

A 60 mJ pulse = 0.06 J = 0.014 cal

This is sufficient thermal energy to heat 1 ml of water by 0.014 °C

But 60 mJ in a microsecond pulse represents a peak power of 0.06/0.000 001 = 60 000 W

The spot size of the laser on the stone is equal to the surface area of the fibre (200 μm radius) = 227 × 0.01 × 0.01 = 0.000 314 cm^2

The peak power density at the stone surface is 60 000/0.000 314 = 190 900 000 W/cm^2

---

portion of the stone surface and made possible by the very high peak power density advisable at the stone surface (Table 8.1).

Animal Experimentation

The pulsed dye laser has been tested in the pig ureter (Watson et al. 1987b). Human urinary calculi were impacted in the proximal ureters, fragmentation with the laser being compared with fragmentation by electro-hydraulic probes. The effect on the ureter of ureteroscopy was compared using a 12Fr and a 10Fr ureteroscope. In all cases where the laser was used there was minimal or no reaction in the surrounding ureter. The use of the electro-hydraulic probe, however, was associated with much more inflammation locally. Thirty pulses at 30 mJ delivered with the laser fibre pushed firmly against the ureteric wall caused a small zone of purpura and penetration of the fibre part of the way through the wall. By contrast, one single discharge of the electro-hydraulic probe too close to the ureteric lumen caused a large perforation in the ureter. Ureteroscopic injury to the ureter was very significant. It was found particularly in the distal third of the ureter and was much more severe after passage of a 12Fr ureteroscope than after the 10Fr ureteroscope. The ureteroscopic injury occurred even though there was no apparent injury at the time of passing the ureteroscope, and its mechanism was not clear. The implications of the study were that the laser is indeed a much more controllable modality for stone fragmentation than is the electro-hydraulic probe. However, perhaps more significant was the impact that the laser might potentially have in miniaturising ureteroscopy, both rigid and flexible.

Q-Switched YAG Lasers

The YAG laser has been developed more than any other laser system for medical applications. It emits at a wavelength of 1064 nm, which is a wavelength at which calculi absorb poorly (Fig. 8.1.). The Q-switched YAG laser with a pulse duration in the region of 10 nanoseconds when focused on a stone surface causes very gradual fragmentation of the stone into very small particles. A plasma is formed with every pulse almost irrespective of absorption, because at these peak power densities a plasma can be formed even in air. The effect on the tissue is to produce minimal ablation.

The initial difficulty is to transmit a pulse of such ultrashort duration via a fibre, because the peak power density within the fibre is close to the damage threshold of quartz. A second problem is that the beam emerging from the distal end of the fibre is divergent. Therefore any separation of the stone from the fibre tip results in a fall-off of the peak power density. However, if the tip is in contact with the stone then it disrupts and ceases to transmit the laser energy. There have been two solutions to this problem (Fig. 8.2.). One solution, developed by Schmidt-Kloiber's team from the University of Graz (Hofmann et al. 1987), is used in the Storz Calculas system. In this the distal end of the fibre is shaped into a lens which limits the usual beam divergence and therefore tends to maintain the power density at the stone surface. The second solution is to place a metal cap between the fibre and the stone, with a small gap between the

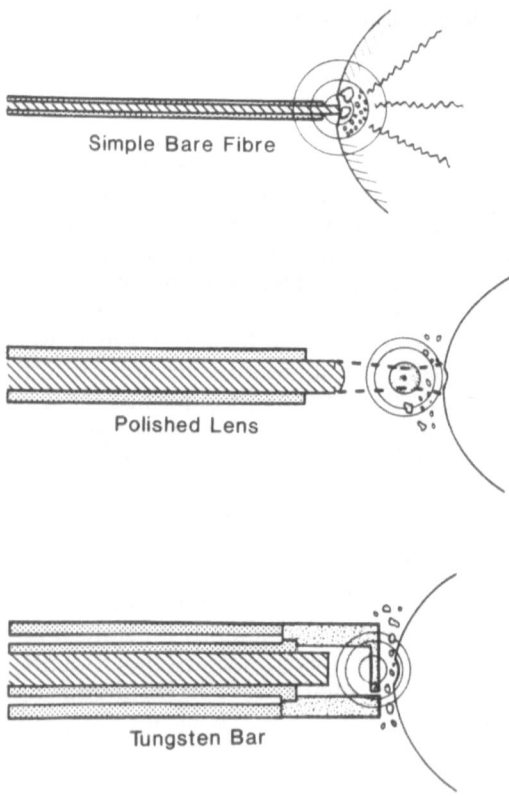

Fig. 8.2. The bare fibre of the pulsed dye system shown alongside the fibres of the two Q-switched YAG systems. (By courtesy of the Institute of Urology.)

fibre and the cap. A shockwave is formed by the action of the laser pulse on the metal and this is transmitted on to the stone.

The Q-switched laser pulses can be delivered via 600-μm core fibres. These fibres are relatively inflexible. Also, both the lens system and the metal cap system are considerably larger in diameter than the simple bare fibre used with the pulsed dye system and cannot, for example, be used via many of the small-calibre flexible ureteroscopes. Both Q-switched laser systems tend to result in a gradual erosion of the stone into small particles, but unfortunately they do not

Table 8.2. A comparison of the pulsed dye and Q-switched YAG laser systems

Parameter	Pulsed dye	Q-switched YAG
Wavelength (nm)	504	1064
Pulse duration (s)	0.000 001	0.000 000 01
Fibre diameter (μm)	200	600
Pulse energy (mJ)	60	30
Peak power density (W/cm²)	190×10^6	1200×10^6
Energy density (J/cm²)	185	12

have any significant action on hard calculi such as those made of brushite or calcium oxalate monohydrate. The metal cap system has been used under X-ray control without endoscopy but with disappointing results, possibly because it is difficult to make direct contact with a stone impacted in the ureter except under vision. The differences between the pulsed dye laser and the Q-switched YAG laser are summarised in Table 8.2.

Using the Pulsed Dye Laser

The pulsed dye laser can be used via miniaturised ureteroscopes. When it was first used clinically the fibre was too small to be used via conventional ureteroscopes and it had to be reinforced by passing it through a catheter. We have therefore campaigned for and contributed to the design of a miniaturised ureteroscope. We suggested incorporating two channels so that irrigation via an independent channel was unaffected by passing the laser fibre. The then novel notion of using fibre-optics in a semi-rigid sheath came from the Candela Corporation. The first prototype was 6Fr and too flexible for insertion above the lower third of the ureter. A subsequent design is 7.2Fr at the tip with re-inforcement to the sheath proximally. This is known as the MiniScope.

Patients and Methods

We have treated 250 patients with one or more ureteric calculi using the pulsed dye laser (Candela Corporation) in combination with miniaturised endo-scopes. The patients ranged in age from 9 to 87 years, 85% being male and 15% female. The calculi had a mean maximum diameter of 11 mm. Fifty-six per cent of the calculi were in the upper third of the ureter and 21% in the middle third. In 18 patients the calculi were multiple.

Ureteroscopy was performed under general anaesthesia. Preoperative anti-biotics were given. The patient's legs were supported in a position rather lower than for conventional cystoscopy. In some patients with lower-third stones, particularly when there was a limitation in abduction of the lower limb, the "scissor position" was adopted in which the ipsilateral hip is flexed and the contralateral hip extended. This allows the operator to stand lateral to the extended thigh and to view from over the leg with a more angled approach into the ureter. The MiniScope was the first instrument to be used in all cases. In all but 15 patients the ureteric orifice was clearly seen and the MiniScope intro-duced with or without first inserting a guidewire a few centimetres up the ureter. In those patients in whom the ureteric orifice could not be identified it was possible to see it using a cystoscope and to then leave a guidewire up that ureter to aid recognition with the MiniScope. No patient required ureteric dila-tation for insertion of the MiniScope into the meatus.

Once the MiniScope was in the ureter the irrigation pressure was reduced to approximately 50 cm of water in order to lessen the risk of flushing the stone proximally. The second instrument channel also allows a degree of free backflow of irrigant which again reduces the intraluminal pressure in the ureter. Whenever there was no clear view of the lumen ahead it was useful to try compression – by means of a hand over the abdomen if the ureter was angling anteriorly or alternatively by lifting the loin anteriorly if the ureter was passing in a posterior direction. A guidewire was frequently useful for pushing the ureteric sidewall away. Another useful technique was to rotate the ureteroscope so that any slight bend in the instrument could be taken advantage of. At no time was there any need for force to advance the ureteroscope. In 10 patients the curves of the ureter were too marked for the passage of the semi-rigid MiniScope and in these the ACMI 8.5Fr actively deflectable ureteroscope was used. The preferred technique was to backload the instrument over a 0.025-inch stiffened guidewire making sure that there were no kinks in the guidewire. When this proved difficult the instrument was introduced through the channel of a 23.5Fr cystoscope.

Laser fragmentation was performed by advancing the fibre until it was touching the stone. A series of bursts of laser energy were then delivered until the stone was fragmented. The process was repeated until all the daughter fragments were reduced to a diameter of 1 mm or less. The laser was disabled (i.e. prevented from delivering laser energy) before removing either the laser fibre or ureteroscope from the patient.

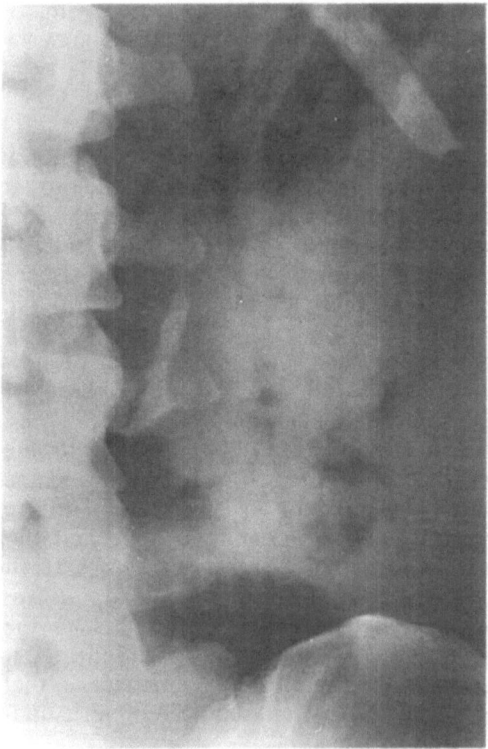

Fig. 8.3. a A ureteric calculus 2.5 cm long and 9 mm wide in the upper ureter. **b** The same patient 24 hours after treatment by laser using the MiniScope. The fragments alongside the double J stent passed and the fragments in the lower pole were treated by ESWL. (By courtesy of the Institute of Urology.)

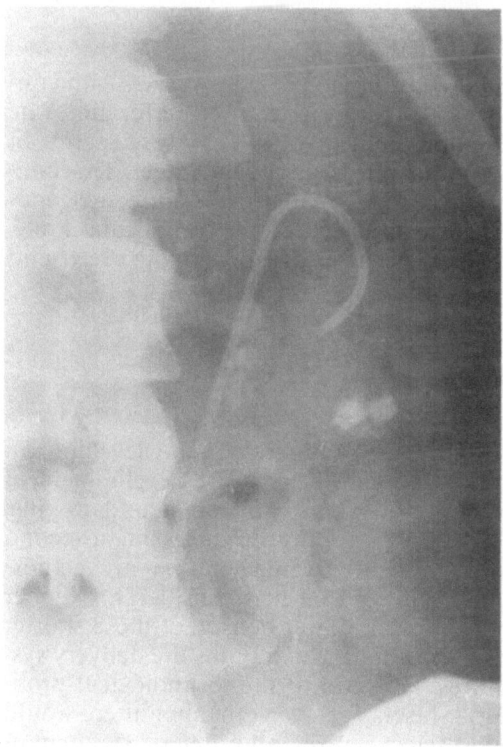

Fig. 8.3b

Results

Using the combination of MiniScope and ACMI flexiscope the ureteric calculi were seen in all but 4 cases. The access failures were due to prostatomegaly in 2 patients and ureteric stricture in 2 patients. In 2 of these failures the stones were nevertheless flushed out of the ureter. The average time taken to reach the stone was 6 minutes using the MiniScope and 38 minutes with the flexiscope. Of the 246 cases where access was achieved all the calculi were successfully fragmented (Fig. 8.3). There were no cases of ureteric perforation and no cases where a needle nephrostomy was required. No patients treated in this way have been known to develop a ureteric stricture. We performed intravenous urograms as a routine 3 months after ureteroscopy for the first 100 patients but the pick-up rate was nil and we have therefore discontinued this unless there are symptoms. There have, however, been other complications. Two patients had a severe pyrexia following therapy with positive blood cultures in one. There were 6 patients who required a repeat procedure to treat a residual fragment which failed to pass spontaneously. In 5 of these a double J stent had been passed in order to keep the ureter clear, but the fragment had descended alongside the stent.

Discussion

In our earlier series (Coptcoat et al. 1987) using the pulsed dye laser with conventional ureteroscopes we reported a 2% stricture rate, a 7% perforation rate and a post-operative nephrostomy requirement of 12%. This was a series in which only 20.3% of the stones were in the upper third of the ureter. This contrasts with our latest series in which the use of smaller-calibre ureteroscopes has improved the efficacy of the procedure and reduced the complication rate, despite the fact that 56% of the stones were in the upper third of the ureter and therefore more liable to complications.

Conclusions

The future of laser lithotripsy lies, I believe, predominantly in the development of cheaper technology to achieve the same parameters. The development of microsecond pulses of green laser light is, however, a challenging undertaking. No solid state laser currently in existence naturally produces microsecond pulses. But shorter pulse duration would only be advantageous if it proved possible to develop fibres to transmit laser energy that had considerably higher damage thresholds: it is the fact that the peak power density of these shorter pulses is so close to the fibre's damage threshold which limits the delivery system to the relatively large-calibre fibres. However, if the technological problems of producing smaller and cheaper lasers are overcome then there would be no reason for lasers to be limited to select centres, and ureteric stone management would become easier and safer for the "jobbing urologist". He cannot refer on all cases of ureteric stone and when he does do a ureteroscopy it is indeed a disadvantage if he has only a large-calibre ureteroscope.

References

Coptcoat MJ, Ison KT, Watson GM, Wickham JEA (1987) Lasertripsy for ureteral stones: 100 cases. J Endourol 1:119–122

Fair HD (1978) In vitro destruction of urinary calculi by laser-induced stress waves. Med Instrum 12:100–105

Hofmann R, Hartung R, Geissdorfer R et al. (1987) LISL: biological effects and first clinical application. Laser 3:247–250

Mulvaney WP, Beck CW (1968) The laser beam in urology. J Urol 99:112–115

Pensel J, Frank F, Rothenberger K et al. (1981) Destruction of urinary calculi by neodymium YAG laser irradiation. In: Kaplan I (ed) Laser surgery IV. Proceedings of the fourth international symposium on laser surgery, Jerusalem. Academic Press, New York

Tanahashi Y, Numata I, Kambe K et al. (1981) Transurethral disintegration of urinary calculi by the use of laser beam. In: Kaplan I (ed) Laser surgery IV. Proceedings of the fourth international symposium on laser surgery, Jerusalem. Academic Press, New York

Teng P, Nishioka NS, Anderson RR, Deutsch TF (1987) Optical studies of pulsed-laser fragmentation of biliary calculi. Appl Phys 42B:73–78

Watson GM, Wickham JEA, Mills TN, Bown SG, Swain P, Salmon PR (1983) Laser fragmentation of renal calculi. Br J Urol 55:613–616

Watson GM, Murray S, Dretler SD, Parrish J (1987a) The pulsed dye laser for fragmenting urinary calculi. J Urol 138:195–198

Watson GM, Murray S, Dretler SD, Parrish J (1987b) An assessment of the pulsed dye laser for fragmenting calculi in the pig ureter. J Urol 138:199–202

Chapter 9

The Future of Lasers in Urology

S. G. Bown and T. A. McNicholas

Paradoxically the future of lasers in surgery generally and in urology in particular may well depend more on improvement in the methods of monitoring the effects of laser techniques than on development of the techniques themselves. That is not to say that major new developments and indeed improvements in what is already available will not be welcome. However, in many respects laser techniques are more precise than the diagnostic and imaging methods that are available. We look forward to a more precise matching of tissue damage to the true extent of the disease than is possible at present, as well as developments in real-time monitoring of what the laser is actually doing to target tissue.

Temperature measurement is at present fairly primitive and most experiments rely on metallic thermocouples with an in-built error due to thermal diffusion down the thermocouple itself. Even though this is probably negligible in most clinical situations it does detract from the overall accuracy of the technique. Recent developments in fibre-optic sensing will allow the accurate measurement of temperatures without this effect. Fine fibre-optic probes will also allow target tissue to be "multiply probed" when appropriate, i.e. when the target is a small, well-defined volume of tissue in close proximity to a vital structure.

Whilst improvements in temperature sensing may well be the most exciting changes in the process of precisely matching tissue damage to the extent of disease, developments in Doppler studies of blood flow and measurements of light intensity within target tissues will contribute to the achievement of the desired precision.

Ultrasound imaging is readily available and lends itself particularly to many urological problems. We have been impressed by the rapid strides that have been made in the quality of the images available and in the resolution of normal from abnormal tissue. Unfortunately this does not mean that the ultimate imaging of the prostate, for instance, has been reached, and it is still disconcerting to find apparently normal images when there is histological proof of abnormality within the gland. There is obviously some way to go before very small tumours, particularly in the prostate, can be accurately defined and we wonder whether this will ever be possible for more diffuse disease. It is of course particularly these small volume cancers to which laser techniques, and specifically methods of interstitial implantation and laser hyperthermia, are most applicable.

The future may allow accurate matching of disease and laser effect to be achieved. At present it is necessary in practice to overtreat a lesion to be sure of the complete destruction of the malignant tissue. This carries the risk of transgression of the laser effect into adjacent vital structures, or indeed into adjacent normal tissue when this is at a premium (as in the poorly functioning kidney). There will obviously be different limits of safety in each organ and between different parts of the same organ and these need to be taken into account when planning treatment.

An accurate indication of the true limits of abnormal tissue, coupled with a true indication of the extent of laser effect, are the twin aims of our current laser research. Ultrasound techniques may have most to offer and we are already beginning to be able to identify the characteristic alterations to tissue architecture resulting from the laser injury. In the future we hope these features will be seen, appreciated and reacted to at the time of treatment when treatment parameters can be altered rather than the information becoming available after treatment when little or nothing can be done about it.

Simply pointing a coagulating laser at a tumour will gradually give way to more precise uses of the laser. We are confident that techniques of implantation of fibres and the use of laser-generated interstitial hyperthermia will play a part in the management of prostate cancer and that the rapidly developing field of photodynamic therapy (PDT) will continue to have a role in the bladder. That role, what is more, will increase once the problems of dosimetry and the choice of the most appropriate photosensitisers have been defined.

The presently available methods of PDT in the bladder, explored by our group and others, suggest at least that with conventional dosimetry there is a significant degree of muscular damage which leads to loss of compliance of the bladder wall with a serious effect on bladder capacity and function. The future may therefore lie in the development of a surface-acting photosensitiser that could be administered intravesically. This would satisfy the twin demands of getting the photosensitiser to the mucosal surface where it is most needed (and where it is least likely to do permanent damage to the bladder wall) and reducing the problems of generalised photosensitisation which up to now have made PDT such an ordeal for the patient. Alternatively and in the meantime generalised photosensitisation is best reduced by using photosensitisers such as the phthalocyanines, that mainly absorb in the red and not elsewhere in the visual spectrum.

In the more distant future applications of PDT outside the bladder will probably grow in importance, particularly where a superficial anti-tumour effect is required, once the appropriate agent to achieve that is available. Multifocal superficial disease in the ureter and pelvicaliceal system are applications that spring immediately to mind. It has always seemed rather a challenge to the urologist that disease in the upper urinary tract has to be treated by wholesale excision of organs whereas, if the same tumour were in the more readily accessible lower urinary tract, it would be treated by local (endoscopic) resection. However, attempts at local resection in the upper urinary tract, whether endoscopic or at open operation, tend to fail with tumour recurrence if there is a widespread "field change" remote from the site of the original tumour. PDT should help in such cases.

The prostate may well become the next focus of attention for PDT, although initially at least it lends itself to interstitial techniques. There is of course no reason why hyperthermic and photodynamic treatments could not both be administered via implanted fibres into the prostate gland; they may indeed have a summating effect. We anticipate that what is left after a very radical endoscopic resection of the prostate may well be amenable to PDT, particularly since a photodynamic effect resulting in tumour tissue death should still leave plenty of relatively resistant connective tissue behind to protect the rectum.

The suggestion that PDT may well have a "collagen sparing effect", as seen in experimental colonic tumours, may revitalise the concept of focal PDT. We have always fought shy of the PDT treatment of deeply invasive tumours on the basis that the degree of necrosis resulting from a full-blown photodynamic effect would impair the structural integrity of the viscus and result in leakage. However, if the collagenous or connective tissue elements of the tumour can be spared then focal PDT treatment might be more relevant in such cases.

Much of the discussion in this book has concentrated on the problems of malignant disease, but it would be wrong to ignore totally the use of the laser in the treatment of benign conditions. The guiding principle must be the same as outlined above: that the laser surgeon must aim to match precisely the type of laser treatment given to the characteristics of the tissue to be treated. For this to be possible, a much more intense study of tissue characteristics and how they relate to laser effect will be necessary.

The comments in this chapter are necessarily speculative - although we hope based on developments of which we are already aware. We make no apology for suggesting some exciting new applications, some of which are bound to fail but others of which may lead on to successful treatments in urology.

Subject Index